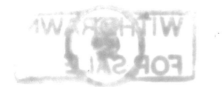

Craniomandibular disorders and orofacial pain

Diagnosis and management

Craniomandibular disorders and orofacial pain

Diagnosis and management

Iven Klineberg, RFD, BDS, MDS, BSc, PhD(Lond), FRACDS, FDSRCS(Eng), FICD
Professor, Department of Prosthetics and Dentistry, University of Sydney, Australia

WRIGHT

Wright
An imprint of Butterworth-Heinemann Ltd
Linacre House, Jordan Hill, Oxford OX2 8DP

 PART OF REED INTERNATIONAL BOOKS

OXFORD   LONDON   BOSTON
MUNICH   NEW DELHI   SINGAPORE   SYDNEY
TOKYO   TORONTO   WELLINGTON

First published 1991

© Butterworth-Heinemann Ltd 1991

British Library Cataloguing in Publication Data
Klineberg, Iven
    Craniomandibular disorders and orofacial pain:
    diagnosis and management.
    I. Title
    617.6

ISBN 0 7236 0989 6

Library of Congress Cataloguing in Publication Data
Klineberg, Iven.
    Craniomandibular disorders and orofacial pain : diagnosis and
    management/Iven Klineberg.
        p.   cm.
    Includes bibliographical references and index.
    ISBN 0 7236 0989 6
    1. Temporomandibular joint—Diseases.   2. Mouth—Diseases.
3. Face—Diseases,   4. Pain.   5. Diagnosis, Differential.
I. Title.
    [DNLM: 1. Diagnosis, Differential.   2. Facial Pain—therapy.
3. Malocclusion—therapy.   4. Temporomandibular Joint Syndrome—
therapy.   WU 140 K65c]
RK470K55   1991
617.5'2—dc20
DNLM/DLC
for Library of Congress

91-26794
CIP

Composition by Genesis Typesetting, Laser Quay, Rochester, Kent
Printed and bound in Great Britain by The Bath Press, Avon

Contents

Foreword

Facial pain remains a challenge to all Dental Specialists despite the dramatic changes in oral disease which currently influence both professional practice and education. Unfortunately the infinite number of remedies and philosophies of pain management bear witness to the worst form of professional fragmentation. This scenario also tells us of the hardline pragmatism which is still regarded by some to be an adequate foundation for treating patients. Such practices will continue until the controlled trial and multidisciplinary management become mandatory in all areas of clinical concern. Iven Klineberg is a Prosthodontist with a renowned research background and a wonderful enthusiasm for scholarship. His book is the first eclectic approach that I know of that combines standard dental management with a detailed discussion of behavioural problems and their medical therapy. Such knowledge is essential for the understanding of a substantial number of patients who are unfortunately often labelled as refractory to treatment. Professor Klineberg has provided the means for all clinicians to understand and help a wide spectrum of pain patients.

Eastman Dental Hospital London   Malcolm Harris

Preface

Craniomandibular Disorders and Orofacial Pain has been written as a clinical manual for dental specialists and generalists. Practical aspects of clinical diagnosis and management of orofacial pain and craniomandibular disorders (CMDs) are covered. The author favours the term CMDs, rather than the commonly used terms temporomandibular (TM) joint dysfunction or myofascial pain dysfunction. The latter terms specify particular aspects of pain and dysfunction which often occur together, but more importantly, these terms do not acknowledge the interrelationships between the cranium, jaw and cervical spine. These interrelationships are important in function and dysfunction and should be acknowledged in management strategies.

Chapter 1 reviews pain and emphasizes the complex psychophysiological basis for it. Chapter 2 reviews diagnosis and management of pain from teeth, jaw muscles and TM joints. Chapter 3 reviews features of the orofacial pain conditions arising from nerves, vessels and a variety of miscellaneous conditions, to emphasize the broad base of knowledge required for differential diagnosis. Chapters 4 and 5 review two important approaches in conservative management for dental practitioners. An Appendix is added as a reference source for the many varied terms used to correctly describe particular conditions.

The incidence of pain and CMDs appears to be either increasing in incidence or represents a significant change in patient demand and therefore direction for dental practice. As a result, there is an increased need by dental practitioners for information concerning diagnosis and management of orofacial pain and CMDs. This change and greater involvement by dentists in this field indicates new responsibilities for them as health care professionals and brings with it the need for a change in practice philosophy and the need for confidence and competence to provide a broad diagnostic base. Change in practice emphasis and demand will continue as community needs alter, and in western countries the earlier emphasis on caries management and restoration of tooth structure is no longer a priority in patient management.

The control of dental caries and the modern conservative approach to tooth restoration has had a profound effect on community needs and focus of dental practice. The changed profile of clinical dentistry now emphasizes the need for other strategies to cope with a broader range of clinical and ethical responsibilities presenting to the dentist. Such changes will encourage the emergence of a discipline for the dental physician.

Dental undergraduate courses are beginning to reflect these changes in emphasis, and will require a broader range of clinical diagnostic skills for the new graduate. Already, an international interdisciplinary committee has made recommendations to the International Association for the Study of Pain on an appropriate syllabus for dental undergraduates in diagnosis and management of orofacial pain and dysfunction.

Sydney, 1990   Iven Klineberg

Acknowledgements

I am grateful to the Editors of the journals and authors listed for their kind permission to reprint the following: *The Dental Clinics of North America* and Dr John Rugh, for permission to use Figure 1.1; *The Mayo Clinic Proceedings* and Dr Frederick Kerr, for permission to use Figure 1.4; *The Australian Dental Journal* for permission to use Figures 4.1, 4.2 and 4.3; *Pain*, for permission to include the Classification of Chronic Pain, Description of Chronic Pain Syndromes and Definitions of Pain Terms; *Cephalgia*, for permission to include the Classification and Diagnostic Criteria for Headache Disorders, Cranial Neuralgias and Facial Pain; and to the Publishers of the texts indicated, for their permission to reprint the following: Plenum Press, for permission to use Figure 1.2; C. V. Mosby Company and *Journal of Prosthetic Dentistry* for permission to use Figure 2.1.

The energy to prepare this manuscript and the motivation and stimulation which was derived from many colleagues with special expertise in this field is acknowledged with gratitude. I am especially aware of the importance of those who influenced and guided my early learning – Emeritus Professor C. H. Graham, formerly Head, Department of Prosthetic Dentistry, University of Sydney; Dr B. D. Wyke, formerly Director, Neurological Unit, Royal College of Surgeons of England; and Professor Emeritus M. M. Ash, formerly Head, Department of Occlusion, University of Michigan.

Many other colleagues have provided stimulation through personal contact and published work and I wish to especially acknowledge Professor M. Harris, Eastman Dental Hospital, University of London (and for his critical comments on the text and his encouragement to complete this work); Professor G. E. Carlsson, University of Gothenburg; Dr A. S. T. Franks, Birmingham Dental Hospital and School (also for his critical comments on Chapter 2); Professor E. Møller, Panem Institute, Copenhagen; Professor J. Lund, University of Montreal; Professor B. J. Sessle, University of Toronto; Professor J. Rugh, University of Texas at San Antonio; Dr J. Marbach, Columbia University, New York; Dr K. Baetz, Prosthodontist, Sydney; Dr R. Hawthorn, Prosthodontist, Sydney; Dr T. Walton, Prosthodontist, Sydney; Dr D. McNamara, Prosthodontist, Perth; and Dr T. Wilkinson, University of Adelaide. Staff in my Department, both full and part-time, who contributed to patient management in my Orofacial Pain Clinic, together with graduate master's degree students in prosthodontics, have been a continual stimulus and motivating force.

My gratitude and special thanks for typing the many drafts and provisional manuscript is extended to my secretaries, Mrs Maree Pearce and Mrs Rebecca Granger for their patience and dedication, and to Ms Prue Wilson for her expertise in preparing the final manuscript and the painstaking work involved in proofing the text.

Finally, and in particular, the support and understanding of my wife Sylvia over many years is acknowledged, together with the patience of Catherine, Stephen, Daniel and Angela who deserved to see much more of their father than was possible.

Chapter 1

Orofacial pain

1.1 Pain perception and transmission
1.1.1 Introduction: Pain – the human experience
1.1.2 Psychology of pain
    Acute and chronic pain
    (a) The emotional-affective system
    (b) Cognitive factors
1.1.3 Physiology of pain
    (a) Pain theories
    (b) Nerve impulse transmission
    (c) Nociceptive pathways
    (d) Modulation of pain
1.1.4 Endogenous control
1.1.5 Acupuncture analgesia
1.1.6 Placebo effects and analgesia

References

1.1 Pain perception and transmission

1.1.1 Introduction: Pain – the human experience

A list of pain terms and definitions may be found in the Appendix (p. 143).

What a human being describes as pain is primarily an emotional experience, not merely the perception of a sensation. This experience is a combination of a pure sensation and the affective reaction (i.e. the suffering aroused by the sensation), and coloured by a variety of visceral reflexes and hormonal changes simultaneously evoked (Wyke, 1976). Thus, the pain presented to the clinician is a complex, highly individual response, and the challenge in diagnosis is in differentiating the physiological and psychological components.

It is commonly regarded in most religions that there is something beneficial in the human experience of pain in the sense that man's moral stature, his personality or his soul is the better for it (Wyke, 1976). This concept is implicit in the word 'pain' in English which has always implied an experience that is chastening. The original English meaning of 'pain' signified punishment, whilst bodily suffering was described by the Latin word 'dolor'. The word 'pain' now implies both of these things.

1.1.2 Psychology of pain

Pleasure and pain are the primary motivators of action, and although psychologists have long been involved in studying the way in which varied motivational conditions (rewards, punishments etc.) influence behaviour, relatively little is known about the fundamental nature of the process of pleasure and pain to which all these motivators refer (Melzack, 1973).

The biological value of pain is often considered to signal tissue damage; however, pain does not always occur after injury, and when it does, the intensity of pain that is felt is not always proportional to the extent of tissue damage. In humans, pain is a complex cultural, cognitive, motivational and emotional experience, dependent upon previous painful experiences, how well we remember these experiences, and our ability to understand the cause of the pain and grasp its consequences (Melzack, 1973).

Thus, pain is a perceptual experience whose quality and intensity is influenced by the unique past history of the individual, by the meaning the individual gives to the pain-producing situation and by his emotional state at the time. Thus, pain can be seen to be a function of the whole individual.

Cultural background plays a fundamental role in pain perception and subsequent reactions, by presenting a code of behaviour which ranges from stoic, where pain is felt only after relatively intense injury as in primitive tribes, to extreme reactions after minor trauma as shown in some modern cultures.

Children are deeply influenced by the attitudes of their parents towards pain, and patterns of behaviour acquired early in life are carried on into adulthood. Attitudes of parents towards dentists are often 'indelibly imprinted' on the minds of their children and can engender fear and apprehension.

Sternbach and Tursky (1965) believe that there are no physiological differences in 'pain threshold'. Regardless of culture there is uniform *sensation threshold*, i.e. the lowest stimulus value at which sensation is first perceived, so that the sensory afferent system subserving nociception is essentially the same in all people. The variation that exists is in *reaction threshold* (this variation is present even in laboratory controlled conditions), and is a reflection of the varying cultural, motivational, cognitive and emotional characteristics of the individual.

Pain is always a psychological event, although the proportional contribution of psychological and physical factors is highly variable. Despite this, it is assumed that pain of 'psychogenic origin' is predominantly or wholly caused by psychological factors, and 'organic pain' predominantly by physical factors. In reality, this is too rigid a view, since psychogenic pain may evoke physical (i.e. organic) pain through peripheral and organ changes associated with the psychogenic response. Nervous system plasticity may result in psychogenic pain evoking the release of neuropeptides and opioides which may cause profound effects of an organic nature.

Pain in the face may be due to local pathology, may be referred to the face from adjacent areas, or may be of psychogenic origin. It should be appreciated that in each case the pain is real to the patient and must be acknowledged as such. Merskey (1984) has reported that 50% of pain of psychogenic origin is experienced in the face and head.

Acute and chronic pain

Acute pain is pain of short duration for which the cause and effect, if readily diagnosed and identified, should allow immediate therapy to be successful.

This contrasts with chronic pain which has been described by Timmermans and Sternbach (1974) as: 'pain of several months duration that resists conventional medical therapies'. Sternbach (1974) has stated further that chronic pain alters the individual's life to such an extent that they may reach a stage where they actually need the pain and cannot live without it. However, this is a punitive view which does not acknowledge the motivation of such patients and in practice is not common.

Thus, in chronic temporomandibular (TM) joint pain, most dentists, becuase of their training and experience in dealing with acute pain and solving relatively simple and easily identifiable cause-and-effect dental situations, consider that there must always be a physical cause to the pain that they should be able to identify and treat. In general, the clinician must acknowledge the patient's affective reaction to the pain and provide both reassurance counselling and physical therapy if indicated.

Whether a pain problem becomes chronic depends in part on the success of the initial therapy, but even more important is the attitude of the first clinician consulted. Moulton (1966) most succinctly identified this situation in a definitive article reporting on emotional factors in non-organic temporomandibular pain and its failure to respond to physical therapy:

The most recalcitrant cases were the patients who had found doctors who promised them complete cures, practitioners who seemed to be sure masters of the situation and who assured them that there was a mechanical way to lift the burden of pain. When such treatment did not give prolonged relief, these patients merely sought another doctor who would hold out hope with a different mechanical method; but as they became increasingly disillusioned and resentful towards dentists, they became less responsive to any treatment.

Pain has been described by Rugh and Solberg (1979) as a 'learned response', the individual's perception of pain being based on experience, memory and learning, which determine the individual response for each person. 'Pain behaviour' is a more appropriate term to denote the individual's general response to pain.

Factors such as stress and emotional disorders such as anxiety or depression, are now known to be major causes of pain, or as modulating influences of so-called organic pain.

The following two descriptions of the pain experience by Sternbach (1968) and Merskey and Spear (1967) emphasize the emotional component of pain:

Sternbach describes pain as 'an abstract concept which refers to:

1. a personal, private sensation of hurt,
2. a harmful stimulus which signals current or impending tissue damage, and
3. a pattern of responses which operate to protect the organism from harm.'

Merskey and Spear state that pain is 'an unpleasant experience which we primarily associate with tissue damage, or describe in terms of tissue damage or both'.

In a comprehensive review, Rugh (1987) states that there is ample experimental evidence confirming a poor relationship between the intensity of a noxious stimulus and the report of and the response to pain, by the patient.

Figure 1.1 is adapted from Rugh (1987) and emphasizes the multi-dimensional nature of pain and links:

1. Peripheral
   – stimuli and the perceptual sensory system resulting in pain behaviour, with
2. Central
   – the emotional-affective system
   – cognitive processes of attention, distraction; beliefs; learning.

The peripheral aspects are described in section 1.1.3, and it is clear that central factors have a direct influence on the peripheral input to either augment or suppress this activity.

(a) The emotional-affective system
Recognition and tolerance of nociceptive (noxious, i.e. have the potential of inducing pain) stimuli are modified by the emotional-affective system

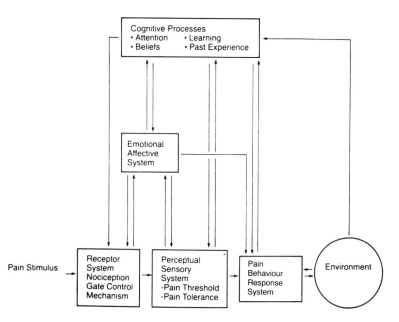

Figure 1.1 A multidimensional model linking pain stimulus with receptor system and perceptual sensory system leading to pain behaviour. The latter is modulated by the emotional affective system, cognitive processes and the environment. Adapted from Rugh (1987)

and by cognitive factors. Anxiety and depression are thought to increase or reduce peripheral nociceptive input via the gate mechanism in the brain stem (see 1.1.3 Physiology of pain), and thereby dramatically modify the patient's perception of pain. Anxiety has the effect of lowering pain thresholds so that anxious individuals experience pain more readily. Depression has been found to influence sensitivity to pain and may increase the patient's pain experience.

(b) Cognitive factors
Cognitive factors (i.e. one's beliefs) may increase or suppress pain, particularly the understanding that the individual has of the pain, its possible cause and its implications.

(i) Attention or distraction Distraction has a powerful influence on reducing or completely masking pain. This is observed most clearly in sport where pain from quite severe injuries, such as a broken finger or dislocated jaw, is not experienced until after the completion of the match. Here the individual's preoccupation with the sporting event suppresses the obvious nociceptive input from the periphery. Once the central influence is reduced, the peripheral factor predominates. Similarly, more deliberate control is possible by actively thinking about and becoming involved in other matters to suppress the pain; or alternatively, focusing on the pain and its implications will enhance the pain experience.

(ii) Beliefs Understanding the cause of the pain and its significance has an important influence and alters pain perception and the individual's ability to tolerate the problem. A non-life-threatening pain caused by a readily identifiable problem such as loss of a dental restoration or dental caries, is

understood by the patient as a readily treatable problem. Pain in an area that does not appear to be so easily treated, e.g. pain in the tongue or head, may appear as a life-threatening disease and the patient's response will be markedly enhanced.

The degree of control is also important in this context. If an individual is able to control the problem, e.g. dietary control in migraine by avoiding specific foods known to cause the pain (such as chocolate, monosodium glutamate, hot dogs etc), then the significance of the pain and its severity are reduced.

(iii) Learning   Learning covers a number of behavioural variations that have been described in different ways:

– Observational Learning or Social Modelling. Bandura (1971) in a comprehensive review concluded that *observation learning* was the main way of acquiring new patterns of behaviour. This is seen particularly well in children, who readily follow the behaviour of other members of the household and particularly their parents. Variations in response are seen in different cultural and ethnic groups where group members provide a model of standards of suffering and whether it should be freely expressed or inhibited.

Craig (1978) discussed similar influences in terms of *social modelling* and reviewed available research in this area. He emphasized the important influence that real experiences or artificial experiences (as in filmed presentations) of pain and injury have on an observer, although there are individual differences in response to another person's injury and suffering. The immediate effect of observing a person in pain can be dramatic and have long-term influences on how the observer subsequently responds to pain.

Craig (1978) suggests that the fear of dental pain is strong enough to avoid visiting a dentist in about 5% of the general population and in about 16% of school children. The current understanding is that such fear is due to unfavourable experiences of other family members, and is thought to be more important than the individual's previously traumatic pain experiences or individual differences in pain tolerance.

– Illness Behaviour. The concept of *illness behaviour* (Mechanic, 1962) describes the ways in which given symptoms may be differently perceived, understood and responded to by different individuals. *Abnormal illness behaviour* is an extension of this concept defined by Pilowsky (1975) as persistent and maladapted perception, evaluation and action in relation to one's health. He describes neurotic and psychotic aspects of abnormal illness behaviour which are readily recognized as hypochondriacal behaviour.

Pilowsky (1978) has described some idiopathic chronic pain as abnormal illness behaviour (see Scott and Humphreys, 1987). In terms of psychodynamic theory, the individual is a 'psychobiological system' where innate and environmental influences interact and must be reconciled in the interests of adaptive function. Pilowsky's neurotic illness behaviour describes pain as a common 'conversion reaction', with a conversion into physical symptoms of repressed emotional conflicts. The characteristic feature is the patient's illness behaviour exhibiting an attitude of dissatisfaction with the pain and a denial of being preoccupied with it or what its cause may be. This strong attitude of indifference also denies any personal problems or any relationship between them and the pain.

In this context Pilowsky associates this conversion with hostile dependency to allow punishment of parents and parental figures (such as clinicians), for repressed sexual drives. His 'psychotic illness behaviour' is described as pain associated with hypochondriacal delusions as part of psychotic depression. In these cases pain is thought to counter (or neutralize) guilt and lessen depression. It is clear that chronic pain of these types (conversion and hypochondriasis) is difficult to diagnose and manage, even in multidisciplinary Pain Clinics. As a result, the term 'abnormal illness behaviour' appears to be the most appropriate one.

Marbach and Lipton (1978) studied aspects of illness behaviour in 170 patients presenting to the Pain Clinic at Columbia University School of Dental and Oral Surgery, with TM joint pain – dysfunction, myofascial pain dysfunction syndrome and atypical facial pain.

Pain was the most common symptom in the face, mouth or neck and occurred in 80% of the patients. The patient's symptoms were significantly related to age and ethnicity, and it appeared that 'factors besides specific signs and symptoms have a significant role in determining if people seek treatment for perceived facial pain and mandibular dysfunction'. These authors concluded that the facial pain problem is a by-product with one of three main origins:

(i) routine dental procedures;
(ii) an illness or;
(iii) an accident,

and is invariably associated with stressful circumstances and coloured by socio-cultural factors. Successful management of these problems requires a sensitive and knowledgeable clinician to relate to the patient in an unthreatening way. Also it is important to offer a management programme that is reasonable and acknowledges the psychological aspects as well as offering appropriate physical therapy.

The assessment of an orofacial pain problem to allow a diagnosis to be made, requires a careful medical and dental history and clinical examination. In order to obtain the appropriate information, a series of questionnaires have been developed and are used together with: (a) other general questionnaires to detect anxiety and depression, and (b) a psychological screening form such as the MMPI (Minnesota Multiphasic Personality Inventory) or a more specific pain assessment, such as the WHYMPI (West-Haven-Yale Multidimensional Pain Inventory – see Kerns, Turk and Rudy, 1985).

The routine Clinical Health Questionnaires designed in the Department of Prosthetic Dentistry, University of Sydney, are shown in Appendix II and are used as follows:

1. A General Information form (1) is completed by patients before the first appointment.
2. A Pain form (2) is completed by patients with craniomandibular pain following the first appointment.
3. A Pain-tension diary (3) is completed by patients where emotional stress is thought to be important in the aetiology.
4. A follow-up form is completed six and/or twelve months after treatment.
5. Specific psychological screening forms are completed by a clinical psychologist.

– Secondary Gain. This is seen where, by maintaining the pain, an individual can gain personal advantage, such as in maintaining the 'sick role' to maximize attention, help and concern of one's family and friends and the like.

1.1.3 Physiology of pain

Noxious stimuli evoke, with short delay, a variety of responses in the individual (Table 1.1), depending partly on the stimulus magnitude, and as well on a number of other factors as previously mentioned, including cultural, cognitive, motivational and emotional factors. These factors result in a variation in response to noxious stimuli in different individuals.

Table 1.1 Reactions to noxious stimuli

Pain
Muscle reflexes – limb withdrawal
               – jaw opening
Startle response
Vocalization
Sweating
Pupillary dilatation
Heart rate increase
Blood pressure changes
Behavioural changes

(a) Pain theories

Ever since von Frey's Specificity Theory (von Frey, 1894), that described specific nerve endings conveying nociceptive information along specific nerve fibres to a specific area in the brain (Figure 1.2), nociceptors have been considered to be free nerve endings. This theory of pain has many shortcomings and does not provide acceptable explanations for many of the complex components of pain. However, single unit electrophysiological studies have confirmed that free endings are nociceptors and certain small diameter fibres are indeed nociceptive afferents, but that nociception is not exclusively conveyed by these fibres.

Noordenbos (1959) described the interaction of large and small diameter fibres and proposed two important developments (Figure 1.2):

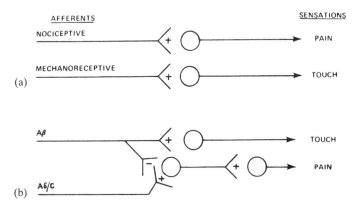

Figure 1.2 Diagrammatic schema of two different pain theories, in which different afferent nerve fibres (on left) involved in particular sensations (on right) are indicated. (a) Specificity theory of von Frey. (b) Sensory interaction theory of Noordenbos (facilitation +; inhibition −). From Dubner, Sessle and Storey (1978)

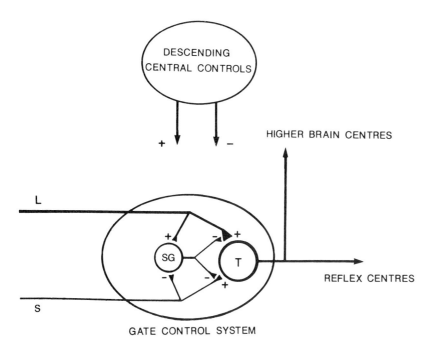

DESCENDING CENTRAL CONTROLS

HIGHER BRAIN CENTRES

L

+   −

SG

−   −

T

+   +

S

REFLEX CENTRES

GATE CONTROL SYSTEM

Figure 1.3 Diagrammatic schema of the principal interactions of peripheral and central influences in transmission of nociceptive afferents as described in the Gate Control theory (Melzack and Wall, 1965). Note that the T-cell is potentially influenced by both large (L) and small (S) diameter fibres from peripheral tissues. However, the information transmitted along large and small fibres is influenced by an interneurone (SG), which for spinal cord afferents is located in the substantia gelatinosa (laminae II and III of the spinal dorsal horn), and for the trigeminal system in nucleus caudalis of the trigeminal spinal nucleus. The interneurone is facilitated (+) by the large fibres and inhibited (−) by the small fibres, and pre-synaptically inhibits the small and large fibre projections to the T-cell. Where there is nociceptive fibre activation, it will facilitate (+) the T-cell and inhibit (−) the SG interneurone. Where there is large fibre activation, as in mechanoreceptor stimulation, the SG interneurone is activated (facilitated, +) and SG projection inhibits S fibres, as well as modulating L fibres. In this way, nociceptive information is blocked, and as a result does not reach the T-cell, whilst large diameter information activates the T-cell. (Adapted from Melzack and Wall, 1965)

(a) interaction of high velocity, large diameter afferents and more slowly conducting small diameter afferents within the central nervous system (CNS), and

(b) this interaction allowed large diameter fibres to inhibit the transmission of small diameter afferents. An understanding of the interaction of nerve fibres of different diameters was an important development, and was a fundamental component of Melzack and Wall's Gate Control theory.

Melzack and Wall (1965) proposed that a gating mechanism exists in the spinal cord substantia gelatinosa to modulate the amount of afferent information transmitted centrally by transmission (or T-) cells (Figure 1.3). The gating mechanism allows inhibition and facilitation to modulate activity of T-cells – large diameter afferent fibres activated by non-noxious influences inhibit T-cells, whilst nociceptive small diameter afferent inputs facilitate T-cells.

In this way T-cell transmission depends on a synthesis or summation of afferent information derived from both nociceptive and non-nociceptive receptors. As well, descending influences from higher brain centres that provide background information concerning cognitive, motivational and emotional components of the sensory experience, also project to T-cells.

This mechanism generated enormous interest in pain research and Kerr (1975) subsequently described a Central Inhibitory Balance theory where neurohistological and neurophysiological investigations allowed a more comprehensive description of the nociceptive and non-nociceptive pathways and interactions. These studies further developed the gate control mechanism. The *nociceptive circuit* (Figure 1.4) involves small diameter afferents whose branches provide both facilitatory and inhibitory

Figure 1.4 Diagrammatic schema of the spinal cord dorsal horn with dorsal root and ganglion (DRG). The principal interactions of large and small diameter afferent fibres as described in the Central Inhibitory Balance theory of pain transmission are shown.

Nociceptive circuit A: s – small diameter afferents; M – marginal neurone; g – gelatinosa neurone; non-nociceptive circuit B: l – large diameter afferents; P – projection neurones.

The layers of the dorsal horn are indicated I, II, III and IV – marginal layer I; substantia gelatinosa layer II, III, magnocellular layer IV.

Nociceptive circuit A: Marginal layer I is where marginal cells (M) are located; these cells are activated (+) by small diameter nociceptive afferents at marginal cell (m) dendrites. They also project to laminae II and III – substantia gelatinosa layers – and activate gelatinosa neurones (g-cells), which provide inhibitory feedback (−) to M-cells. M-cells project their axons to the spino-thalamic tract.

Non-nociceptive circuit B: Large diameter afferents project to layer III to excite gelatinosa neurones (g) and dendrites of projection neurones P-cells, located in magnocellular layer IV. The g-cells project powerful inhibitory feedback to marginal neurones.

It can be seen that both circuits activate g-cells, but the large fibres activate a much greater number of g-cells. As the g-cells inhibit the M-cells, the greater the number of g-cells activated, the greater the M-cell inhibition. This is balanced by s-fibre activation of M-cells, and so a balance of s and l fibres influences projection of nociceptive information reaching M-cells. This is the basis of the 'inhibitory balance' theory. From Kerr (1975) with permission

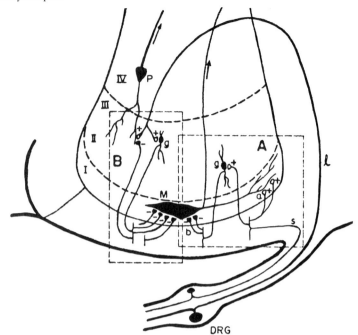

influences to marginal neurones. The latter act as nociceptive transmission cells. The *non-nociceptive circuit* describes large diameter primary afferents that enter the spinal cord and synapse with projection cell dendrites (P-cells) and inhibitory interneurones (gelatinosa or G-cells); the latter have inhibitory influences on marginal cells. Both afferent fibres activate inhibitory interneurones, but the large diameter non-nociceptive fibres activate a greater number at different levels of the spinal cord.

Thus the idea of central inhibitory balance arose between small and large diameter inputs, where a dominance of large fibre inhibitory influences results in an inhibitory balance controlling the output of marginal (T-cells) cells. The nucleus caudalis of the spinal tract of the trigeminal nerve blends with substantia gelatinosa of the spinal cord, and nociceptive afferent connections in the trigeminal system have been shown to have many similarities with spinal cord nociceptive pathways.

(b) Nerve impulse transmission

Nerve impulse transmission is a function of nerve fibre diameter and the presence or not of myelin sheathing of the nerve fibre. The larger the nerve fibre diameter, the faster the velocity of impulse transmission.

Myelin lamellae from Schwann cells cover all myelinated nerve fibres and where adjacent Schwann cell lamellae approximate there is a gap of varying size, termed the node of Ranvier. Impulse transmission occurs by membrane depolarization and ionic exchange across the membrane in areas not sheathed in myelin. In myelinated nerve fibres, depolarization occurs at successive nodes of Ranvier (so-called saltatory conduction), whilst with non-myelinated fibres membrane depolarization progresses along the entire nerve fibre membrane. As a result, myelinated nerves conduct more rapidly than unmyelinated fibres.

The more rapidly conducting A-delta fibres are thought to be responsible for 'first' or 'fast' pain, and the more slowly conducting C-fibres for 'second' or 'slow' pain. These different pain responses are important in pain from structures more distant in the body than the head. As the distance travelled from orofacial structures is very short, these two types of pain sensation are not clearly identifiable in orofacial pain.

However, the two fibre types are also responsible for different pain quality:

1. A-delta fibres are thought to be responsible for acute, sharp and well localized pain; and
2. C-fibres are responsible for dull, more diffuse or poorly localized, aching pain.

A classification of nerve fibres is shown in Table 1.2. It can be seen that nociceptive information may be transmitted by A-delta and C-fibres, but these two fibre types also convey information from thermoreceptors, low threshold mechanoreceptors and pre- and post-ganglionic autonomic fibres respectively.

It is apparent from this classification that the different types of fibres are associated with different peripheral receptor systems and effector systems, and are thus involved in different sensory-motor activity. The larger nerve fibres, A-alpha fibres for example, convey afferent (i.e. sensory)

Table 1.2 Classification of peripheral nerve fibres (developed from Sessle, 1981)

Fibre type		Diameter (μm)	Conduction (m/sec)	Receptor afferent	Effector efferent
Roman Numeral	Greek Letter				
I	A–α	12–21	70–120	Muscle spindle –primary afferent Golgi tendon organ	α-Motoneurone axons to skeletal muscle
II	A–β	6–12	35–70	Muscle spindle –secondary afferent Low threshold mechanoreceptor	
	A–γ	2–8	12–48		γ-Motoneurone axon to muscle spindle
III	A–δ	1–6	2.5–35	Low threshold mechanoreceptors Thermoreceptors Nociceptors	
	β	1–3	2.5–15		Preganglionic autonomic fibres
IV	C	0.4–1.2	0.7–1.5	Low threshold mechanoreceptors Thermoreceptors Nociceptors	Postganglionic autonomic fibres

information from large complex peripheral mechanoreceptors, such as muscle spindles and tendon organs; alpha fibres also provide efferent (i.e. motor) connection via motoneurones to motor end plates of skeletal muscle.

Smaller nerve fibres have different afferent receptor associations and different efferent influences.

In each peripheral receptor system an adequate stimulus will evoke a generator potential in the receptor nerve ending which is responsible for triggering an action potential in the afferent fibres. This is conveyed centrally to contribute to an appropriate response.

(c) Nociceptive pathways

(i) Peripheral projections – Nociceptive afferent pathways from the orofacial area.

Sensory afferent information from the face and mouth is relayed along branches of the sensory root to cranial nerves V, VII, IX, X and cervical nerves C1, C2, C3 to the brainstem nuclear complex. Afferent fibres branch on entering the brainstem to project to the main sensory nucleus and as well to nucleus caudalis of V (Dubner, Sessle and Storey, 1978). It is in the latter region of V that the gating of nociceptive afferents occurs. Also, descending influences from the cortex and other regions of the CNS have the capability of modifying this afferent input, before trigemino-thalamic transmission.

(ii) Central projections   Projections from the nucleus caudalis occur along two distinct pathways to the thalamus.

The first is the bulbothalamic tract (an extension of the spinothalamic tract). The relatively few synaptic connections along this pathway suggest that this route is responsible for subserving 'first' or 'fast' pain, which is the first sensation felt and is sharp in character and well localized.

The secondary pathway is the reticulothalamic pathway involving projections to the limbic system. Collateral projections from the bulbothalamic tract project to the brainstem reticular formation and via a series of interneurones project along a multisynaptic pathway, conduct more slowly, and are probably associated with 'second' or 'slow' pain. Connections from reticular formation to parts of the limbic system are important, as limbic structures provide the neural basis for the potent motivational and affective components of pain.

Projection from thalamus to cortex: Projection from different thalamic nuclei to specific areas of the cerebral cortex is dependent upon the existence of a certain level of activity in thalamic transmission neurones, which is influenced by the amount of large diameter mechanoreceptor afferent inputs reaching nucleus caudalis and then thalamic nuclei, from coincident stimulation of mechanoreceptors and nociceptors.

The sensory discriminative (perceptual) component of pain is provided by transmission neurones in the posteroventral nucleus of the thalamus projecting to the parietal and inferior paracentral regions of cortex. This allows recognition of location and the physical nature of the painful experience. Both sides of the face project to each area of cortex (Wyke, 1976).

The motivational and affective component of pain is provided by projections from the dorsomedial nucleus of the thalamus which receives inputs from the reticular formation and from bulbothalamic tracts via intralaminar nuclei from the posteroventral thalamic nucleus. Projection to the frontal cortex (orbital region) provides the unpleasant, emotional aspects of pain, i.e. the 'second' pain component. This projection is part of the limbic system and is the phylogenetically older system, operating in conjunction with the newer bulbothalamic projection pathway.

It is the involvement of this part of the frontal cortex that separates pain from other special sensory experiences – such as vision, hearing and touch, because it provides the unique, unpleasant quality that disrupts ongoing behaviour and thought, and requires immediate attention. The removal of this component of intractable pain, by dividing these thalamocortical connections in prefrontal leucotomy (Freeman and Watts, 1950), has confirmed this association.

The memory of pain is evoked by thalamocortical projections to the temporal cortex in the ventromedial parts, where memory of past painful experiences is stored. Previous experiences of pain have a profound influence on subsequent pain experiences.

Also, projections to hypothalamus from the reticular formation, and descending thalamic-hypothalamic projections evoke the variety of visceral-hormonal reflex effects (Wyke, 1976) (involving cardiovascular, gastrointestinal and respiratory systems), that characterize the total experience of pain.

(d) Modulation of pain

Peripheral modulation of nociceptive afferent information arises by the effects of large diameter mechanoreceptor afferents simultaneously evoked. This large fibre modulation may be enhanced by a variety of procedures including; rubbing and massage of the affected site; acupuncture needling, transcutaneous neural stimulation; and the like.

Cutaneous hyperalgesia may follow nerve trauma, such as occurs with post-herpetic neuralgia, where viral damage to nerve cells of large diameter afferents occurs, resulting in a reduction of their usual inhibitory effects, until they regenerate. With increasing age, a progressive degeneration of large diameter myelinated afferents results in a reduction in their central inhibitory effects and may be partly responsible for a reduced pain tolerance in elderly people.

Central modulation occurs in the nucleus caudalis of the trigeminal nucleus, the thalamic nuclei and the cerebral cortex. Projections from the lateral reticular formation (LRF) relay to interneurones in the nucleus caudalis resulting in presynaptic inhibition of orofacial nociceptive afferents. This descending inhibitory influence occurs together with large diameter interactions from orofacial tissues and represents another gating mechanism controlling the central projections of nociceptive afferents. The level of LRF inhibition varies and may be augmented or inhibited by a

Table 1.3 Reticular formation (adapted from Wyke, 1976)

1   Caudal (posterior) inhibitory projections
     (Relieves intensity and awareness of pain by presynaptic inhibition in nucleus caudalis)

1.1 Augmented by – distraction, concentration
                  – hypnosis
                  – certain drugs: amphetamines,
                                   chlorpromazine (Largactil),
                                   diazepam (Valium).
                                   morphine and its derivatives,
                                   carbamazepine (Tegretol), and
                                   diphenylhydantoin (Dilantin)

1.2 Reduced by certain drugs – barbiturates (Nembutal, Seconal)

2   Rostral facilitatory projections
     (Cortical activation and so increased intensity and awareness of pain)

2.1 Augmented by – anxiety
                  – alcohol in small amounts
                  – caffeine
                  – certain drugs: dextroamphetamines (Benzedrine),
                                   cannabis (Marijuana), and
                                   lysergic acid diethylamide (LSD)

2.2 Reduced by – emotional tranquillity
                – sleep
                – alcohol in large amounts
                – hypocarbia (by hyperventilation), and
                – certain drugs: Meperidine (pethidine)

variety of medications and drugs and by varying levels of excitability (Table 1.3).

A variety of neurochemicals is associated with both descending inhibitory pathways and inhibitory circuits within the spinal cord to modulate nociception, the complexity of which is only now becoming apparent.

In a comprehensive review, Dubner (1985) reports on the following neurotransmitters released from descending brainstem pathways:

1. Substance P may be released from descending excitatory pathways, or be released locally from spinal cord interneurones where it may have excitatory or inhibitory effects;
2. Serotonin (5-HT) originates as an inhibitory neurotransmitter from neurones of descending inhibitory pathways and acts by postsynaptic inhibition directly on spinothalamic neurone excitability and enhancing arousal behaviours; and
3. Noradrenaline is released from descending pathways to inhibit trigeminothalamic and spinothalamic neurones or via dorsal horn interneurones.

Within the spinal cord and presumably the trigeminal nucleus, some neurochemicals acts as conventional excitatory and inhibitory neurotransmitters, e.g. gamma aminobutyric acid (GABA) and glutamate respectively, whilst others do not produce changes in membrane permeability, but act as modulators to enhance or reduce the action of other neurotransmitters. A diversity of neurochemicals within the spinal cord are available for modulation of nociceptive afferent information (Dubner, 1985): Encephalin is released from descending inhibitory axons and from dorsal horn neurones, which have been shown to inhibit nociceptive thalamic projection neurones. GABA is released by spinal interneurones to inhibit thalamic projection neurones. Other inhibitory neurotransmitters acting within the spinal cord include substance P, cholecystokinin and somatostatin.

It is apparent that as well as controlling nociceptive afferent transmission, the many different neurochemicals present in the spinal cord have various roles and contribute to the plasticity of response of individuals to nociception.

Rostral reticular activation of the cerebral cortex varies with the level of excitability in the reticular formation and this provides an alerting mechanism for cortical neurones. Descending corticofugal influences on transmission cells in the trigeminal nuclear system also occurs, and the level of corticofugal inhibition depends on the level of cortical activation. These effects appear to increase the individual's awareness of the area of nociceptive stimulation.

It is apparent that modulation of nociceptive information occurs peripherally and centrally. The latter involves complex interrelationships between reticular inhibitory and activating systems, descending corticothalamic, corticobulbar (to brainstem trigeminal nuclei) and other descending inhibitory influences, as well as complex interconnections for modulation at the segmental level of spinal cord and trigeminal spinal nucleus.

1.1.4 Endogenous control

It was discovered by chance that electrostimulation of certain parts of the brain, specifically the periventricular and periaqueductal regions, produced analgesia in animals and man. Morphine was known to produce analgesia, and both these analgesic effects were shown to be inhibited by naloxone, a specific morphine competitor. Thus it became apparent that a morphine-like substance was implicated in electrostimulation, and the search for an endogenous opiate began in many research centres.

Studies employing autoradiography of brain sections (Snyder, 1977) showed that the distribution of opiate receptor sites parallels the paleospinothalamic pain pathway, and a high density of opiate binding sites is present in all parts of the limbic system that mediate emotional behaviour. Micropipette injections have identified specific opiate receptor sites and confirmed the presence of a natural morphine-like transmitter substance. Such a substance has been identified and called encephalin. It has been shown that encephalins are neurotransmitters of specific neuronal systems in the brain that mediate the integration of sensory information to do with pain and emotional behaviour.

The pituitary adenohypophysis produces, amongst other things, ACTH and β-lipoprotein, the latter being the immediate precursor of β-endorphin. Both ACTH and β-endorphin are secreted simultaneously by the pituitary as a response to acute stress (Akil *et al.*, 1984), and the regulating mechanism involved in secretion and biosynthesis is identical. Beta-endorphin given intravenously in appropriate amounts to rats causes analgesia of up to one hour, whilst larger doses may result in a variety of effects including: rigidity, loss of corneal reflex, loss of righting reflex, and changes in body temperature. It has been shown that endorphin is involved in a number of physiological processes such as pain perception, pain tolerance, temperature regulation, eating, learning, sexual behaviour and central regulation of the cardiovascular system and respiration (Goldstein, 1976).

Nociceptive modulating systems derived from within the CNS project as descending inhibitory fibres to the spinal grey matter and the trigeminal spinal nucleus. These descending inhibitory systems arise from the nucleus raphé magnus (NRM) and LRF (Fields and Basbaum, 1978). Axons from NRM are inhibitory seratonergic fibres (releasing inhibitory neurotransmitter 5-HT) and those from LRF are inhibitory noradrenergic fibres (releasing inhibitory neurotransmitter noradrenaline) (Basbaum, 1984).

Inhibition in the spinal grey matter or trigeminal spinal nucleus may occur by postsynaptic inhibition of projection neurones and/or presynaptic inhibition of nociceptive afferents (Dubner, 1985). Which mechanism occurs depends on the particular spinal cord cells with which the descending inhibitory fibres synapse (there is presumably a similar mechanism in the trigeminal system). Activity of cells of origin of the descending inhibitory fibres in the NRM is controlled by the hypothalamus and the limbic system.

The natural opiates suggested the key to a non-addictive opiate with powerful analgesic properties. Animal tests, however, showed the encephalins to be highly addictive, suggesting that we are addicted to our own internal opiates. This has generated much interest and there is no doubt that this opiate receptor represents a new site for potent pain relieving drugs.

1.1.5 Acupuncture analgesia

Systematic investigation of acupuncture in animals and man has been in progress for the last decade, in an attempt to understand and explain its varied effects and in particular the mechanism of acupuncture analgesia (for review, see He, 1987). Much of the mystery associated with acupuncture and the purported traditional need to balance the energy source of the body, may be explained on the basis of Western neurophysiology (Westerman *et al.*, 1989).

The most confusing aspect of acupuncture analgesia is that needling specific skin points results in analgesia in areas remote from the needling. However, needling an affected area also results in analgesia at the site (Price *et al.*, 1984). It is likely that this effect arises as a result of the stimulation of large diameter afferents, the effects of which dominate at the segmental level and block nociceptive afferents by the gating mechanism described by Melzack and Wall (1965). Le Bars, Dickenson and Besson (1983) explain the analgesia of specific areas from needling specific skin points remote from the area by a mechanism termed diffuse noxious inhibitory control – DNIC. DNIC is considered to involve endorphin secretion (Mayer, Price and Rafii, 1977), and descending inhibitory seratonergic pathways evoked by the needling. This second stimulus (the needling) results in enhanced centre-surround inhibition (Le Bars, Dickenson and Besson, 1983; Westerman *et al.*, 1989) which in turn blocks transmission of nociceptive afferents already evoked.

Centre-surround inhibition arises in the spinal cord and brainstem by the action of descending modulating pathways (from the periaqueductal grey) which are tonically active, and which under normal circumstances reduce the background afferent activity affecting the transmission cells. This will have the effect of enhancing a noxious stimulus. In the case of acupuncture, the needling is a second noxious stimulus, which is enhanced by the effects of centre-surround inhibition, whilst the first noxious stimulus (the nociceptive input evoking the pain) is reduced. This results in analgesia. Thus, centre-surround inhibition develops as a result of the needling noxious stimulus which evokes a combination of peripheral and central inhibitory mechanisms, resulting in analgesia. The observed difference in responsiveness to acupuncture may be associated with endogenous endorphin secretion and the availability of opiate receptors.

Although acupuncture analgesia is possible, there is a strong cultural association with its reported effectiveness, and it is generally not used alone for surgical procedures if conventional anaesthetic agents are available. In multidisciplinary management of chronic pain, acupuncture is valuable; however this writer agrees with the strong reservation and absence of scientific data expressed by Westerman *et al.* (1989) in relation to the use of acupuncture in the treatment of disease.

1.1.6 Placebo effects and analgesia

About 35% of patients report marked relief of pain after being given a placebo (Beecher, 1972). This remarkably powerful effect in no way implies that the pain is not real. It indicates, however, a powerful contribution of suggestion to the perception of pain, and emphasizes the significance of the emotional component of pain. Placebo itself seems to be based partially on the unwritten contract between clinician and patient, which states that the former is going to do everything possible to relieve the patient's suffering. Gardner and Licklider (1959) found that intense auditory stimulation (white noise) suppressed the pain produced by restorative dental treatments and extractions, and they termed this effect 'audio-analgesia'. The effects of audio-analgesia on some patients was dramatic, but did not always occur – the machine worked well for some people but not on others.

This created enormous interest, but following controlled tests (Melzack, Weisz and Sprague, 1963) it was found that 'audio-analgesia' was only effective if it was accompanied by strong suggestion. Clearly then, this approach would be effective in the hands of clinicians with strong personalities and a strongly persuasive manner, able to convince their patients that they would feel less pain.

Alternatively, it would be less successful in the hands of those with a more cautious approach. Patients of course varied in their susceptibility also and this fact interacted with the clinician's approach. The enthusiasm for use of audio-analgesia fell rapidly as it was seen not to block pain in an 'all or none' manner; it was in effect a placebo response.

Until the identification of endogenous opiates (endorphins), the mechanism of placebo action was not understood. Placebo analgesia and narcotic analgesia appear to have a similar mechanism, and people who respond to placebos obtain significantly more relief from narcotic analgesia. If placebo-induced analgesia is mediated by endorphins, then naloxone, a specific opiate antagonist, would block its effects. In a clinical study (Levine, Gordon and Fields, 1978) employing a placebo, it was found that naloxone, when administered with morphine, increased pain to a greater extent than the placebo; it also brought the mean pain rating to the same level as that of placebo non-responders.

This convergence suggests that most if not all the analgesic effect of a placebo is naloxone-reversible. It would thus appear that endorphin activity accounts for placebo analgesia, since naloxone causes a greater increase in pain in placebo responders than in non-responders; and previous administration of naloxone reduces the probability of a positive placebo response.

References

Akil, H., Watson, S. J., Young, E. *et al.* (1984) Endogenous opioides: Biology and function. *Annual Review of Neuroscience*, **7**, 223–255

Bandura, A. (1971) In *Psychological Modeling: Conflicting Theories* (ed. A. Bandura), Aldine/Atherton, Chicago, pp. 1–62

Basbaum, A. I. (1984) Functional analysis of the cytochemistry of the spinal dorsal horn. In *Advances in Pain Research and Therapy* (eds H. L. Fields, R. Dubner and F. Cervero), Raven Press, New York, Vol. 9, pp. 149–175

Beecher, W. K. (1972) The placebo effect as a non-specific force surrounding disease and the treatment of disease. In *Pain: Basic Principles, Pharmacology, Therapy* (eds R. Janzen, W. D. Keidel, A. Herz and C. Steichell), Georg Thieme, Stuttgart

Craig, K. D. (1978) Social modeling influences on pain. In *The Psychology of Pain* (ed. R. A. Sternbach), Raven Press, New York, pp. 73–109

Dubner, R. (1984) Specialisation in nociceptive pathways: sensory discrimination, sensory modulation, and neural connectivity. In *Advances in Pain Research and Therapy* (eds H. L. Fields, R. Dubner and F. Cervero), Raven Press, New York, Vol. 9, pp. 111–137

Dubner, R., Sessle, B. J. and Storey, A. T. (1978) *The Neural Basis of Oral and Facial Function.* Plenum Press, New York, p. 18

Fields, H. L. and Basbaum, A. I. (1978) Brainstem control of spinal pain-transmission neurons. *Annual Review of Physiology,* **40**, 217–248

Freeman, W. and Watts, J. W. (1950) *Psychosurgery in the Treatment of Mental Disorders and Intractable Pain.* Thomas, Springfield, Ch. 10, pp. 353–374

Gardner, W. J. and Licklider, J. C. R. (1959) Auditory analgesia dental operations. *Journal of the American Dental Association,* **59**, 1144–1149

Goldstein, A. (1976) Opioid peptides (endorphins) in pituitary and brain. *Science,* **193**, 1081–1086

He, L. (1987) Involvement of endogenous opioid peptides in acupuncture analgesia. *Pain,* **31**, 99–121

Kerns, R. D., Turk, D. C. and Rudy, T. E. (1985) The West-Haven-Yale multidimensional pain inventory (WHYMPI). *Pain,* **23**, 345–356

Kerr, F. W. L. (1975) Pain. A central inhibitory balance theory. *Mayo Clinic Proceedings,* **50**, 685–690

Le Bars, D., Dickenson, A. H. and Besson, J. M. (1983) Opiate analgesia and descending control systems. In *Advances in Pain Research and Therapy* (eds J. J. Bonica, U. Lindblom and A. Iggo), Raven Press, New York, Vol. 5, pp. 341–372

Levine, J. D., Gordon, N. C. and Fields, H. L. (1978) The mechanism of placebo analgesia. *Lancet,* **ii**, 654–657

Marbach, J. J. and Lipton, J. A. (1978) Aspects of illness behaviour in patient with facial pain. *Journal of the American Dental Association,* **96**, 630–638

Mayer, D. J., Price, D. D. and Rafii, A. (1977) Antagonism of acupuncture analgesia in man by the narcotic antagonist naloxone. *Brain Research,* **121**, 368–372

Mechanic, D. (1962) The concept of illness behaviour. *Journal of Chronic Diseases,* **15**, 189–194

Melzack, R. (1973) *The Puzzle of Pain.* Penguin Books, New York, pp. 100–103

Melzack, R., Weisz, A. Z. and Sprague, L. T. (1963) Strategems for controlling pain: contributions of auditory stimulation and suggestion. *Experimental Neurology,* **8**, 239–247

Melzack, R. and Wall, P. D. (1965) Pain mechanisms: a new theory. *Science,* **150**, 971–979

Merskey, H. (1984) Too much pain. *British Journal of Hospital Medicine,* **31**, 63–66

Merskey, H. and Spear, F. G. (1967) *Pain: Psychological and Psychiatric Aspects.* Baillière, Tindall and Cassell, London, p. 21

Moulton, R. E. (1966) Emotional factors in non-organic temporomandibular joint pain. *Dental Clinics of North America*, (Nov.), 609–620

Noordenbos, W. (1959) *Pain.* Elsevier, Amsterdam, p. 182

Pilowsky, I. (1975) Dimensions of abnormal illness behaviour. *Australian and New Zealand Journal of Psychiatry,* **9**, 141–147

Pilowsky, I. (1978) Psychodynamic aspects of the pain experience. In *The Psychology of Pain* (ed. R. A. Sternbach), Raven Press, New York, pp. 203–217

Price, D. D., Rafii, A., Watkins, L. R. and Buckingham, B. (1984) A psychophysical analysis of acupuncture analgesia. *Pain,* **19**, 27–42

Rugh, J. D. (1987) Psychological components of pain. *Dental Clinics of North America,* **31**, 579–594

Rugh, J. D. and Solberg, W. K. (1979) Psychological implications in temporomandibular pain and dysfunction. In *Temporomandibular Joint: Function and Dysfunction* (eds G. A. Zarb and G. E. Carlsson), C V Mosby, St Louis, pp. 240–268

Scott, J. and Humphreys, M. (1987) Psychiatric aspects of dentistry. *British Dental Journal,* **163**, 81–84

Sessle, B. J. (1981) Pain. In *Oral Biology* (eds G. I. Roth and R. Calmes), C V Mosby, St Louis, p. 9

Snyder, S. H. (1977) Opiate receptors and internal opiates. *Scientific American,* **236**, 44–56

Sternbach, R. A. (1968) *Pain: a Psychophysiological Analysis.* Academic Press, New York, p. 12

Sternbach, R. A. (1974) *Pain Patients: Tracts and Treatment.* Academic Press, New York, pp. 52–78

Sternbach, R. A. and Tursky, B. (1965) Ethnic differences among housewives in psycho-physical and skin potential responses to electric shock. *Psychophysiology,* **1**, 241–246

Timmermans, G. and Sternbach, R. A. (1974) Factors of human chronic pain: an analysis of personality and pain reaction variables. *Science,* **184**, 806–808

von Frey, M. (1894) Die Gefuhle und ihr Verhaltris zu den Empfindungen. Beit z Physiol des Schmersinnes. Berichte uber die verhandlung d konigl sachs. Leipzig, Gesellschaft d Wissenshaften

Westerman, R. A., Bogduk, N., Mendelson, G. *et al.* (1989) *Acupuncture.* National Health and Medical Research Council Monograph. Canberra: NH and MRC, 1–84

Wyke, B. D. (1976) Neurological aspects of the diagnosis and treatment of facial pain. In *Scientific Foundations of Dentistry* (eds B. Cohen and I. Kramer), Heinemann Books, London, pp. 278–299

Further reading

Elton, D., Stanley, G. and Burrows, G. (1983) *Psychological Control of Pain*, Grune & Stratton, Sydney

Holzman, A. D. and Turk, D. C. (1986) *Pain Management. A Handbook of Psychological Treatment Approaches*, Pergamon Press, New York

Mumford, J. M. (1976) *Toothache and Orofacial Pain*, 2nd edn, Churchill Livingstone, Edinburgh

Sternbach, R. A. (1978) *The Psychology of Pain*, Raven Press, New York

Chapter 2

Aetiology, diagnosis and management of craniomandibular pain

2.1 Introduction
2.1.1 Terminology

2.2 Pain from teeth
2.2.1 Pulpal innervation
2.2.2 Dentinal sensitivity
2.2.3 Clinical assessment
 (a) General
 (b) Cracked tooth syndrome
 (c) Referred pain from teeth
 (d) Phantom dental pain and dental causalgia
 (e) Phantom bite

2.3 Psychogenic pain
2.3.1 Introduction
2.3.2 Clinical features
 (a) TM joint dysfunction
 (b) Phantom tooth pain
 (c) Atypical facial pain
 (d) Hypochondriasis
 (e) Monosymptomatic hypochondriacal psychosis
2.3.3 Management

2.4 Muscle pain
2.4.1 Introduction
2.4.2 Acute muscle pain
 (a) Mechanical trauma
 (b) Muscle fatigue
 (c) Reflex muscle hyperactivity
 (d) Clinical signs
2.4.3 Chronic muscle pain
 (a) General features
 (b) Myofascial pain dysfunction syndrome
2.4.4 Management
 (a) General
 (b) Clinical approach

2.5 Temporomandibular joint pain
2.5.1 Introduction
 (a) Craniocervical aspects
 (b) Signs and symptoms
 (c) Clinical signs

2.1 Introduction

The management of orofacial pain involves procedures that may be employed routinely by dental clinicians. The diagnostic features and management methods appropriate for structured and psychogenic pain originating in teeth, jaw muscles, temporomandibular joints and craniocervical structures are described. As pain may also arise from other sites in the head and neck, the management depends on careful differential diagnosis.

A comprehensive history, a careful clinical examination and correlated special tests are essential requirements (Table 2.1). A standardized approach employing detailed history and examination forms (see also Chapter 1) allows a systematic analysis of pain problems, and minimizes the likelihood of omitting important details.

Table 2.1 Orofacial pain and dysfunction

1. History
    Medical
    Dental

2. Orofacial Examination
    Clinical occlusal analysis
    Cranial nerve examination

3. Special Tests
    Pulp test of individual teeth (CO_2 pulp tester preferred to
       electric pulp tester)
    Study casts articulated
      Laboratory occlusal analysis
    Radiographs
    OPT
    Intra-oral – bitewing and periapical
    TM joint
      Standardized transcranial – joint position
      Plain tomography
      Computed tomography
      Arthrography – internal joint derangement
      Magnetic resonance imaging
    Other
      TM joint arthroscopy
      EMG – jaw reflexes
      Jaw movement

Two important features of pain management must be recognized:

1. The therapeutic effect of reassurance – so-called 'placebo-response', is a highly significant factor. Approximately 45% of patients may show a positive placebo response. This fact must be developed by the clinician adopting a sympathetic and explanatory approach to each pain problem.
2. Pain syndromes have a cyclical history with natural exacerbations and remissions. For this reason short-term 'success' of a particular treatment may have coincided with the beginning of a period of remission, in which case exacerbation of symptoms will occur after a variable period.

Thus success of a particular form of treatment requires long-term follow-up, and can only be fully evaluated in a double-blind, controlled trial.

There is currently considerable confusion concerning the aetiology and management of many craniomandibular pains. The problem arises because of the involvement of the teeth, jaw muscles and TM joints – areas considered specifically dental territory, and to be managed by dental means. This has involved primarily mechanical approaches such as occlusal splints, occlusal adjustment and jaw repositioning, which relate directly to undergraduate dental training with its traditional emphasis on mechanical treatment in restorative dentistry.

Since dental caries is now well controlled in many countries through the use of fluoride in reticulated water supplies, in dentifrices and topical applications, together with a marked improvement in oral hygiene awareness and routine, there is now time for management of other dental needs. Unfortunately, dental education is slow to catch up with community needs, and the emphasis on mechanical therapy remains the cornerstone of treatment-based dental education.

Generally, teaching and training of the management of craniomandibular pain is often absent or not well developed. The result is that dental graduates are poorly trained in background knowledge and diagnostic and management methods for craniomandibular dysfunction and pain. This results in a dental population with a need for information, who are readily influenced by clinicians promoting mechanical and electronic instrumentation, often in conjunction with commercial interests and without the necessary scientific research data to justify their claims of usefulness in diagnosis and management of craniomandibular dysfunction and pain.

This has led to the development of two distinct schools of thought – one that promotes physical treatment (splints etc.), and the other that promotes medical management (muscle relaxant, antidepressant medications etc.). The differences are clearly derived from different clinical training and thus a different understanding of the aetiological mechanisms and how to deal with them. This is well illustrated in the dialogue between Professors Berry (prosthodontics) and Harris (maxillofacial surgery), reported in the *British Dental Journal* (1985).

It is clear that in order to bridge this gap, it is necessary to accept that:

1. Specialized pain clinics attract the more intractable pain problems;
2. Pain of psychogenic origin is a reality to be dealt with in the appropriate way; and
3. Functional disorders of the craniomandibular system may be managed with dental therapy.

2.1.1 Terminology

A number of terms have been used to describe similar conditions ever since Costen drew the attention of clinicians to the possibility of a physical dysfunction of the jaw joint with a variety of associated symptoms. The terms commonly used are listed below:

Costen's syndrome (Costen, 1934)
Temporomandibular joint pain dysfunction syndrome (Schwartz, 1955)
Atypical facial pain (Rushton, Gibilisco and Goldstein, 1959)
Functional disturbances (Olsson, 1969)
Myofascial pain dysfunction (Laskin, 1969)
Masticatory pain – dysfunction (Bell, 1973)
Facial arthromyalgia (Harris, 1974)
Mandibular dysfunction (De Boever, 1979)
Temporomandibular disorders (Griffiths, 1983)
Craniomandibular disorders (McNeill *et al.*, 1980; McNeill, 1983; Nordic Meeting of Stomatognathic Physiology, 1986; Wänman, 1987)

The variety of terms suggests that the mechanism and aetiology of the clinical conditions are poorly understood. However, the term 'craniomandibular disorders' more correctly describes the close interrelationship of cranial and mandibular structures both in function and dysfunction. These relationships are important in diagnosis and management of these problems.

Craniomandibular disorders (CMDs) are defined by Wänman (1987) as: 'Functional impairment of the masticatory system, signs and symptoms of mandibular dysfunction, associated headache and facial pain.'

2.2 Pain from teeth

Dental pain refers specifically to pain arising from tooth pulp and/or dentine and is usually described as acute discomfort. When the tooth pulp is involved by traumatic injury or dental caries, inflammation stimulates pulpal nociceptive afferents, and the unyielding walls of dentine forming the root canal prevent swelling, so that intrapulpal pressure increases with a further augmentation of pain. Pain is invariably the major pathophysiological response experienced from the pulp.

2.2.1 Pulpal innervation

The pulp contains a profuse innervation of A-delta (small myelinated – $1–4\,\mu m$) and C (unmyelinated – $<1\,\mu m$) – fibres, which are involved in nociception and sympathetic efferent control of pulpal blood vessels. The number of nerve fibres reaching the pulp primarily through the root apex varies in different teeth and continues to increase after eruption. Johnsen, Harshbarger and Rymer (1983) found that human premolars contained as many as 1800 nerve fibres following eruption but that this number decreased with age. This is compatible with progressive degeneration of nerve fibres throughout the body with increasing age and the reduced sensitivity of teeth in the older adult.

The A-delta and C-fibres in the pulp conduct nociceptive information differently (see Chapter 1, Section 1.1.3(b) for details).

Närhi, Hirvonen and Hakamäki (1982) used single fibre electrophys-iological recordings in the dog and found that:

1. A-delta fibres responded to dentinal stimulation that would normally cause pain associated with cavity preparation, and rapid thermal stimulation of the tooth, whilst C-fibres were not activated.
2. C-fibres were evoked by slow thermal stimulation which did not stimulate A-delta fibres. It would appear that A-delta fibres are responsible for dentinal pain and C-fibres for pulpal pain.

Nerve fibres generally accompany blood vessels into the pulp as a neurovascular bundle and do not branch until they reach the coronal pulp. As myelinated nerves approach dentine they lose their myelin and branch repeatedly, forming a plexus or network of fibres adjacent to the odontoblast layer called the subodontoblastic plexus of Raschkow (Fearnhead, 1963; Trowbridge, 1986). Fearnhead identified the presence of nerve fibres entering dentine tubules and was doubtful about their role in subserving dentinal sensitivity.

Electronmicroscopic studies (Frank, 1968) showed nerve fibres in the pulpal end of some dentine tubules in close association with odontoblast processes. Although it was considered that communication between dentinal nerve fibres and the odontoblast process may provide the means of mechanoreceptor transduction in dentinal sensation (Anderson, Hannam and Matthews, 1970), this has not been confirmed (Byers and Matthews, 1981).

Trowbridge (1986) and Gunji (1982) describe fibres from the plexus of Raschkow:

1. Extending through the odontoblast layer and ending on odontoblast cells in an expanded ending, so-called marginal fibres;
2. Other fibres loop back towards the pulp and have a beaded appearance and these expanded areas contain mitochondria and other organelles (Harris and Griffin, 1968);
3. Other fibres branch freely in the predentine layer providing a dense innervation of the predentine, where about 25% of human premolar teeth contain nerve fibres as reported by Lilja (1979);
4. Some fibres enter the dentine tubules and extend a short distance and a few may extend as far as 10 µm (Gunji, 1982);
5. Pulpal innervation is densest beneath cusp tips and in this location many nerves extend into dentinal tubules (Byers and Dong, 1981);
6. Närhi *et al.* (1987) showed that mechanical procedures, e.g. drilling and air drying dentine, injured the odontoblast layer and the structural relationship of pulpal nerves of the pulp–dentine border. However, intradental nerves retained their responsiveness to dentine stimulation and this alteration was presumably reversible.

It is clear from the above that the dentine tubules have no nerve fibres over their outer two-thirds, their penetration into the tubules occurring for 0.1–0.2 mm into the pulpal ends. This limited presence of nerve fibres in a proportion of dentine tubules and the fact that communication between odontoblast and nerve fibres has not been satisfactorily demonstrated, indicates that another mechanism must be responsible for dentinal sensation.

2.2.2 Dentinal sensitivity

Brännström (1963) presented an alternative explanation for dentine sensitivity in his hydrodynamic theory, which may also explain the common clinical observation that the dentino-enamel junction is the most sensitive part of dentine. It is considered that fluid flow along dentine tubules provides the transduction necessary to evoke related nerves in the pulp. The odontoblast process extending through the pulpal one-third of the dentine tubule will be traumatized during cavity preparation or affected by deep carious breakdown. In any event there would be loss of fluid from the tubule and fluid flow provides a mechanical stimulus for evoking a pulpal afferent response.

In a recent review, Trowbridge (1986) strongly supports the mechanism of fluid flow along dentine tubules as described by Brännström originally, as being responsible for dental pain. Trowbridge described the normal fluid flow occurring along a pressure gradient causing fluid to flow through dentine tubules and through minute pores in the enamel. With cavity preparation and removal of enamel, fluid flow is much greater. As dentine tubules are tapered towards the enamel, varying from 2.5 μm at their pulpal end to 0.8 μm at the dentino-enamel junction, fluid flow is greater from cut tubules at the dentino-enamel junction, since the effect of capillarity is enhanced by the smaller diameter (Garberoglio and Brännström, 1976) at the cut end.

With exposure of dentine tubules during cavity preparation and particularly during desiccation from air blasts commonly used for drying dentine, fluid flow from dentine tubules is enhanced. Rapid flow of fluid outwards has been proposed by Brännström and Åström (1972) as the critical component of the electromechanical transduction required for stimulation of pulpal nerve endings located at the pulp–dentine junction. The mechanical effect of fluid flow appears to be the adequate stimulus to evoke a generator potential in the adjacent nerve endings and action potential propagation along nociceptive afferents in the pulp.

Thermal stimuli to human teeth have been shown by Trowbridge *et al.* (1980) to evoke pain before the temperature changes reached pupal afferents and that fluid flow in dentine tubules was the likely means of transduction, i.e. thermomechanical stimulation. These authors proposed that heat applied to the tooth surface would produce an expansion in dentine fluid and so a linear movement which may be sufficient to stimulate adjacent pulpal nerves.

Pulpal inflammation

Acute inflammation in the pulp changes pulpal physiology and causes pulpal nerves to become hypersensitive. This causes a condition of hyperalgesia (i.e. an increased response to a stimulus which is normally painful), and may also produce allodynia (i.e. evoking pain by a stimulus that would not normally produce pain) (see Appendix for terminology).

This situation arises for two important reasons: firstly the presence of inflammatory mediators released during the inflammatory process (such as bradykinin and 5-hydroxytryptamine) appears to lower the threshold of nerve endings, i.e. produce an increased sensitivity to appropriate stimuli; and secondly the change in tissue fluid dynamics in the inflammatory response, which characteristically results in inflammatory fluid with swelling or increased pressure in enclosed body spaces such as within joint capsules and tooth pulps. The increase in pulpal pressure is another possible mechanism for increased responsiveness of pulpal tissue.

The amount of inflammation may have a bearing on the graded sensitivity observed clinically where pulpitis may vary from an acutely distressing condition to one of minimum discomfort.

Clinical experience suggests that the dentino-enamel junction is the most sensitive zone of dentine. There is no neural mechanism to account for this effect, i.e. nerve endings do not extend throughout dentine nor are nerve fibres present in the majority of dentine tubules, and odontoblast processes extend only through the pulpal one-third of the dentine. The hydrodynamic effect of fluid flow from cut dentine tubules, with a rapid change in fluid dynamics stimulating pulpal afferents, is the most likely mechanism. Also, the presence of a greater density of fine tubules at the dentino-enamel junction may also contribute to the heightened sensitivity.

As previously reported, capillarity is enhanced in small diameter tubules, and the increased number of small tubule branches may account for a more rapid fluid outflow and so a greater sensitivity at the dentino-enamel junction.

2.2.3 Clinical assessment

The exact mechanism of dentinal sensitivity is not yet fully understood; however, from a clinical viewpoint certain features should be considered in differential diagnosis:

(a) General

Pain originating in dentine or pulpal tissue remains the commonest cause of orofacial pain in most populations, although there are regional differences where the effect of fluoride has dramatically reduced the incidence of caries. In such populations orofacial pain involving the jaw muscles and jaw joints has achieved a relatively higher incidence.

Despite this careful clinical and radiographic assessment of teeth, periodontal and gingival tissues, it is essential to confirm the presence of a dental pain problem. Particular difficulties may arise in the diagnosis of a 'cracked' tooth.

(b) Cracked tooth syndrome

This condition is not uncommon and involves adult posterior teeth mainly. It is a condition that is poorly recognized as a possible cause of orofacial pain arising from teeth and must be considered as a potential cause of pain in differential diagnosis.

A number of terms have been used to describe this condition including:

split tooth syndrome
incompletely fractured tooth
cuspal fracture
coronal fracture
split-root syndrome
dentinal crack syndrome

(i) Aetiology A variety of clinical situations have been correlated with cracked teeth. The following are the most commonly observed aetiological factors:

– teeth subjected to a traumatic incident;
– teeth under heavy occlusal loads, particularly associated with tooth clenching;
– heavily restored teeth with weakened transverse and triangular cusp ridges;
– root-filled teeth are an increased risk; and
– older teeth become more brittle, particularly older root-filled teeth.

(ii) Differential diagnosis (Tables 2.2, 2.3) Symptoms may vary from difficulty or vague and mild discomfort on chewing fibrous, tough or granular foods, to pain of varying severity and duration. The varying symptoms are related to the location and size of the defect in the tooth.

In vital teeth a small incomplete fracture of the crown will give discomfort, whilst a larger incomplete fracture will cause low-grade pain and discomfort. Complete fracture reaching the pulp chamber will give acute pain either with loading of the cusp to cause minute separation of the tooth segments, or with the release of loading and subsequent aggravation of pulpal tissue. As the crack becomes more extensive it may cause sudden, sharp, distressing pain of short duration on the affected side.

The crack may involve the crown only and present as an incomplete fracture either vertically or obliquely. An oblique fracture may be

Table 2.2 Vital cracked tooth

Symptoms
– intermittent acute pain
– provoked by cold and chewing tough/grained food
– may refer pain to ipsilateral face

Examination
– tooth vital
– not generally sensitive to percussion
– bruxofacets on cuspal inclines
– tooth usually heavily restored
– ice always evokes pain but heat only where crack is extensive
– crack sometimes detected with aid of transillumination and staining after removal of restoration
– tooth sensitive to dental procedures without local anaesthesia
– radiograph negative

Table 2.3 Non-vital cracked tooth

Symptoms
– intermittent aching pain
– pain referred to ipsilateral teeth and face
– varied stimuli provoke pain

Examination
– tooth non-vital, may be root filled
– sensitive to percussion on buccal, lingual, occlusal surfaces
– may be sensitive to palpation
– not sensitive to cold or heat
– crack may be detected with aid of transillumination and staining
  after removal of restoration
– radiograph may show lateral periapical rarefaction, other
  periodontal defect, extent of root filling, post etc.

Periodontal assessment
– crack involving root may have infra bony pocket
– if pocket depth is >5 mm, tooth extracted or root resected

supragingival or extend subgingivally. Vertical fractures may involve the pulp and if it extends into the root will evoke acute pain.

In non-vital, teeth if the crack extends to the root there will be periodontal pain and the progressive development of an infra bony pocket adjacent to the split, which may discharge into the gingival crevice with acute exacerbations.

Brännström (1986) has identified bacteria located within the crack allowing their migration and their products to the pulp. This contributes to pulpal hypersensitivity and subsequent inflammation.

(iii) Clinical signs   A number of clinical signs are indicative of teeth that may be split. Invariably the patient will not be able to identify the specific tooth involved, although they will be able to highlight the area in the arch where the problem is located.

1. The patient will have developed an altered chewing pattern to avoid biting hard on particular teeth, especially with fibrous, tough or granular foods. The clinician must ask specifically about this development.
2. There may be a history of a 'masticatory accident', such as unexpected contact with a hard object with eating after which time the patient became aware of avoiding sensitivity in one area of the mouth (Rosen, 1982; Swepston and Miller, 1986).
3. Specific sensitivity to cold such as ice applied to the tooth cusp:
   a small crack will result in short pain (< 1 min);
   a larger crack will result in pain of longer duration;
   cracked teeth are often insensitive to heat, unless the lesion is extensive or has been present for a long time.
   Examination should reveal one or more of the following:
4. A tooth in heavy occlusion – note heavy bruxofacets particularly indicating excessive horizontal loading;

5. A heavily restored tooth crown with an underfilled occlusal surface allowing opposing tooth cusps to extend deeply into the occlusal surface and leading to a wedging effect on the already weakened tooth crown;
6. A non-vital tooth that has been root filled and excessively instrumented;
7. A root-filled tooth with post and core, especially where the post extends deeply into the root and mechanical preparation has removed excessive tooth structure;
8. A root-filled tooth where the core does not incorporate a reinforcing collar to fully surround and support the prepared root face; and
9. The presence of a deep pocket surrounding a root-filled tooth that develops acute inflammation with suppuration and discharge through the gingival crevice. It is common for the deep pocket to develop at the site of the split root only, and for the remaining gingival crevice to be of standard depth for the particular tooth.

(iv) Radiographs   Radiographs may not show the crack but will indicate:

1. The extent of cavity preparation and the vulnerable areas of the tooth,
2. The extent of root canal instrumentation,
3. The extent of post preparation,
4. The presence and location of pins.

In some cases there may be a periapical radiolucency but the pathognomic sign is a unilateral radiolucency along the lateral aspect of the root adjacent to the fracture.

(v) Management involves supporting the tooth to avoid further extension of the crack (Table 2.4):

Vital teeth – replace restoration to support tooth cusps and avoid undercontouring. With restoration removed, transillumination may identify the crack. Adjust opposing plunger cusps and horizontal loading of cusps in lateral excursions.

Non-vital teeth – root-canal therapy followed by a post and core. Care must be taken to support adequately the root face with a 'collar extension' (Rosen, 1982) so that the full crown supports the root and avoids excessive lateral loading.

Where possible, ensure that lateral guidance on anterior teeth will reduce excessive horizontal loading of posterior teeth.

(c) Referred pain from teeth
Referral of pain from teeth to superficial facial tissues may occur and overlap with pain referral zones from jaw muscles. Provocation testing by biting on a firm object (Krogh-Poulsen and Olsson, 1969) to provoke a differential increase in pulpal or muscle pain will help to confirm the existence and location of a split tooth.

(d) Phantom dental pain (or atypical odontalgia, idiopathic periodontalgia) *and dental causalgia*
Diagnosis of these two conditions is often difficult and confusing, and reports in the literature do not differentiate their specific and characteristic

Table 2.4 Treatment of cracked tooth

VITAL TOOTH

Incomplete fracture
– relieve occlusion, remove plunger cusps
– sedative dressing
– replace restoration, restore centric stop at correct occlusal height

Oblique fracture
– supra gingival
  – relieve occlusion
  – sedative dressing
  – replace restoration
– subgingival
  – relieve occlusion
  – sedative dressing
  – restore with crown

Vertical fracture
– relieve occlusion
– root canal therapy
– crown to reinforce tooth; avoid excessive horizontal forces in
  lateral excursions
– extraction may be indicated

NON-VITAL TOOTH

No furcation involvement
– root canal therapy
– may need post and core – must reinforce root
– full crown

Furcation involvement
– root canal therapy
– root resection
– full crown
– extraction may be indicated

---

features. Phantom dental pain has been described (Marbach, 1978b) as a deafferentation pain with a mechanism similar to phantom limb pain (Melzack, 1971; 1973). Deafferentation pain of dental origin is more correctly termed dental causalgia and so-called phantom dental pain is more correctly termed atypical odontalgia.

(1) Phantom dental pain – atypical odontalgia   Such pain presents in one or a number of teeth with long standing acute pain. There may be a history of extensive and unsuccessful dental treatment which may have included restorative and endodontic treatments, followed by extraction. Such treatments may provide short-term relief but the pain invariably returns with greater severity. A large number of such patients have a history of depressive illness marked by anxiety and stress (Harris, 1974; Rees and Harris, 1978). Harris (1991, personal communication) describes the following features that differentiate phantom dental pain or atypical odontalgia:
(a) It may arise in vital, unfilled and non-damaged teeth;
(b) It may remit spontaneously or in response to medication with tricyclic or monoamine oxidase inhibitor drugs, which suggests that it does not have

have a structural basis. Such medication is effective even when the condition is of many years duration;

(c) It may migrate to different tooth quadrants, which further differentiates this problem from nerve damage or neuroma formation;

(d) It often arises simultaneously or sequentially with atypical facial pain or craniomandibular disorders, and therefore may have some common mechanism;

(e) It may follow the cessation of anti-depressant therapy in a depressed patient;

(f) It was formerly provoked by the drug 'Serpasil' which was known to deplete the central nervous system of 5-hydroxytryptamine and cause depression;

(g) It is a common cause of litigation, particularly when it involves a vital unrestored tooth – the tooth may be prepared for a sedative dressing and then restored, followed by root canal therapy, and finally extraction – but the pain persists.

(2) Dental causalgia (or deafferentation pain)   Pain may arise following the loss of nerve elements such as occurs in endodontic therapy, tooth extraction, or intra-oral surgical procedures, each of which is responsible for trauma to peripheral branches of the trigeminal nerve.

There may be either a peripheral or a central neural mechanism or a combination of both (Gregg, 1978).

Possible peripheral mechanisms

Following a traumatic nerve injury, such as that accompanying pulpal avulsion or tooth extraction, peripheral nerve degeneration occurs. This is seen in the peripheral nerve after one week, and in the central processes and second order neurones after approximately four weeks (Gregg, 1971). Whether regeneration occurs depends on a number of factors, and even if some regeneration of individual fibres occurs, it may not be complete.

This is particularly so with large diameter fibres where regeneration of myelin sheaths is often incomplete. Larger nerve fibres and larger ganglion cells are more severely affected by nerve injury than small fibres and cells.

Deafferentation pain is unremitting, is felt at the site of nerve injury, and is accompanied by burning, boring or pressure sensations that may become diffuse. It is relieved often by local anaesthetic infiltration at the site of injury, the analgesic effect of which may long outlast the period of anaesthesia. It will not respond to any form of occlusal, muscle or restorative therapy, nor to medication.

Peripheral nerve trauma thus may lead to aberrant nerve repair. Peripheral post-traumatic neuromas may develop at the site of the peripheral lesion (i.e. intra-alveolar branches to tooth pulp and periodontal tissues following root canal therapy and/or tooth extraction).

Such development at the site of regeneration may allow ephaptic transmission (i.e. communication between nerve fibres) which is suggested as a possible mechanism for tactile hypersensitivity and burning sensation (Gregg, 1978). It has also been shown that even after long-term regeneration, the relationship between large and small fibres in terms of pain modulation may not be re-established (Bray and Aguayo, 1974; Howe, 1983).

The modulation of nociceptive afferents by larger fibres will change, as larger fibres are affected more severely than small fibres, so that the 'inhibitory balance' or 'gating' of nociceptive afferents will be different. As smaller diameter C-fibres will be affected less severely than the larger A-delta fibres, the increase in 'second' or 'slow' pain sensations (dull, diffuse, aching and burning pain sensations), may occur in this way.

The aetiology of phantom phenomena is not understood, however peripheral and central neural mechanisms have been proposed. The possible peripheral mechanism has been described above; however, surgical excision of neuroma formation, peripheral nerve section (e.g. neurectomy) or nerve section within the brainstem (gasserian rhizotomy) or thalamus, is not always effective in management of phantom pain (Melzack, 1971).

Possible central mechanisms

Central nervous system mechanisms have been proposed (see Melzack, 1971, 1973 and Marbach, 1978b for review):

– Psychological mechanisms contribute to phantom phenomena which may be triggered by emotional disturbances and relieved by hypnosis and psychotherapy (Melzack, 1971).

– Central biasing: Altered gating of nociceptive afferent information from the site of tooth loss, has been proposed by Melzack (1971, 1973) because of initial loss of nociceptive and larger diameter afferent influences. The central influences would then have a greater effect on transmission neurones (see Gate control theory, Chapter 1, Section 1.1.3 and Figures 1.3 and 1.4). This is suggested as an explanation for the change in the 'inhibitory balance', that under normal circumstances modulates nociceptive afferent transmission.

Following regeneration of damaged nerves the possibility of aberrant neuronal communication, associated with nerve sprouting and ephaptic transmission, will increase the projection of peripheral information, i.e. produce hyperactivity, and further alter central biasing.

It is likely that mechanisms such as those proposed by Melzack are responsible for phantom pain. Also, altered sensations associated with missing teeth, particularly the 'feeling' that the teeth were distorted in shape and increased in size, has been reported (Marbach, 1978a).

More recently, Howe (1983) successfully treated a case of deafferentation pain in a 45-year-old man following a motor cycle accident with severe injuries to chest and brachial plexus, but no spinal cord damage. The pain in the affected right arm was aching, burning, cramping, lancinating, and varied in severity but was always present. Following unsuccessful treatment with medication and following neurophysiological testing, dorsal horn coagulation eliminated the sensory phenomena.

Howe (1983) proposed that dorsal horn neural plasticity following brachial plexus avulsion was responsible for the phantom phenomena, where aberrant repair led to the deafferented second order neurones becoming 'reafferented' by low threshold primary afferents from adjacent dermatomes. This mismatch of primary and second order neurones (or aberrant repair) was thus responsible for the clinical features of light touch producing pain (hyperpathia) in the phantom and the denervation hypersensitivity. Similar mechanisms may also exist in dental causalgia.

(e) Phantom bite

Phantom bite has been described by Marbach (1976, 1978a). This condition does not present as pain, but is included to assist diagnosis. This is a psychiatric condition which develops as a result of irreversible dental treatment. Where there are significant changes in tooth position or shape, there may follow changes in perception of intercuspal tooth contact (i.e. the bite). The patient is aware of and becomes preoccupied with this change in sensation or 'loss' of their original 'bite', and seeks further treatment to regain their pre-treatment situation. Repeated dental treatment does not restore this 'loss', but adds to the patient's frustration and despair.

Marbach (1976) hypothesizes that this change in the bite is of a similar nature to phantom limb with profound alteration in proprioception associated with lost tissue and in the patient's understanding and acceptance of this change. This clinical condition may be termed hypochondriacal psychosis or neurosis and requires medical management – see Chapter 5, Section 5.2.4 for further information.

The condition of phantom bite may be more simply understood as occlusal hyperawareness or an iatrogenic dysproprioception (Harris, 1991; personal communication).

Although it is considered that this type of problem has a psychological basis, there may also be a physical component.

It is known that during development, motor skills are acquired at different rates and to varying degrees. Some children and adults have relatively poor motor skills, as evidenced by a relatively poor ability at sport (particularly ball games), handwriting and an awkwardness with locomotion and general motor performance; they are slow to learn new motor skills. Alternatively, others are gifted at sport and other motor skills and learn new skills rapidly and to a high degree of precision.

In terms of motor control of jaw movement, the same range of abilities may exist in re-learning jaw movements following major changes to the contact surfaces of the teeth. Those patients who suffer from phantom bite may have generally poor motor skills.

Precision of jaw position and movement appears to be related to peripheral feedback of jaw movement and tooth contact through cerebellum to motoneurones. It has been shown that periodontal and probably other (mucosal, periosteal) mechanoreceptors have a direct (i.e. without the presence of interneurones) connection, ending as Mossy fibres on granular cells of the cerebellar cortex (Elias *et al.*, 1987; Taylor *et al.*, 1987). This suggests the importance of such peripheral feedback in movement control and especially at tooth contact. These authors propose that muscle spindles in jaw closing muscles provide general feedback to motoneurones to monitor length changes associated with jaw opening and closing. However, this must be calibrated or modulated by an additional feedback system to provide kinaesthetic perception and precision. The periodontal (mucosal and periosteal) mechanoreceptors appear to have this role. The plasticity of the cerebellum in relearning a new jaw position at tooth contact and/or movement path to and from tooth contact may show great variation, in the same way as general motor skills vary. This may be responsible for some patients not readily adapting to changes made to tooth form and guidance. Thus, there may be a physiological as well as a psychological component to the problem of phantom bite.

Clinical studies are needed to investigate this hypothesis, and to allow a more appropriate management of these complex clinical problems.

(ii) Management of phantom tooth pain (atypical odontalgia)   Conventional dental treatment is not effective. This is apparent by the commonly presenting history of phantom tooth pain where root-canal treatments for adjacent teeth followed by extraction of teeth progressively has occurred. Only short-term relief is produced after each procedure, and with the return of symptoms the treatment is repeated on an adjacent tooth. An entire arch of teeth may be lost in this way, with the pain remaining unabated.

Medical management has been suggested by Marbach (1978b), Harris (1974) and Rees and Harris (1978) with the minimum of dental intervention. The following (Harris, 1991; personal communication) supercedes the recommendation of Rees and Harris (1978).

– Tricyclic antidepressant (nortriptyline)
 dose: 10–20 mg nocte for six weeks and increasing to 50–100 mg if necessary.
 Symptom relief should be apparent after one to three months, but occasionally if there is no response a mono-amine oxidase inhibitor (phenelzine – Nardil) may be used.
 dose: 15 mg t.d.s. (the last dose at 4 pm) increasing to 30 mg mornings and 15 mg b.d.

2.3 Psychogenic pain

2.3.1 Introduction

Regional psychosomatic disease is usually well accepted when the response to stress or an emotional illness can be seen or measured. Eczema, asthma, or even irritable bowel, are examples where the physician would not hesitate to eliminate a psychogenic aetiology. Unfortunately, psychogenic orofacial pain has no signs and worse still, the actual disturbance in function is not understood. Hence the clinician can only recognize the pattern of presentation, seek a history of adverse life events and evidence of an emotional response, but must accept that the pain is real and arises from neuropeptide release in blood vessels or adjacent to nerve endings.

In a contemporary understanding of illness, there is increasing awareness of the interplay between psychological and organic factors, and that physical symptoms may be exaggerated by psychological stress or be due to an underlying psychological disorder (Scott and Humphreys, 1987).

The dentist's awareness of these factors is crucial to their successful management of many pain problems.

One difficulty for dentists to overcome is the fact that their patients see them as being primarily concerned with the mouth and teeth and not general health, and that their clinical skills are highly developed but mechanically based. Secondly, approximately 90% of patients suffer pre-treatment anxiety when visiting a dentist (Scott and Humphreys, 1987) which is unrelated to education or illness in general.

One factor may be a previous traumatic dental incident and/or pain, particularly in older people, whose previous experiences of dental treatment were often unhappy ones (Franks, personal communication, 1989). Kent (1985) reported that in relation to recalling past experiences of dental pain, anxious patients described more pain at subsequent appointments than was previously described. This is in keeping with the hypothesis that patients' memory of pain experience is reconstructed with time and becomes consistent with their level of anxiety.

In management of craniomandibular pain a clear distinction must also be made by the dentist between acute and chronic pain. Although a majority of acute pain problems involving the teeth, jaw muscles and TM joints may be managed by a variety of dental procedures, it must be appreciated that most chronic pain problems are not related to the occlusion and their management cannot be approached by traditional dental treatments.

The presence of the 'vulnerable pain person' has been described by Harris in the editorial of the *British Dental Journal* (1984; **156**, 155) which proposes that: 'In childhood such patients may suffer abdominal or ear pain; in adolescence TM joint pain, migraine and dysmenorrhoea; and later, headache, neck and back pain . . .' and possibly also pruritis, irritable colon and non-allergic rhinitis.

A number of authors (Berry, 1969; Marbach and Lipton, 1978; Greene, Olson and Laskin, 1982; Feinmann and Harris, 1984a; Dworkin and Burgess, 1987; Scott and Humphreys, 1987), have described such features in their chronic pain patients.

Feinmann and Harris (1984a) emphasized an important feature of chronic orofacial pain that was previously described by Moulton (1955) and Lupton (1969), but apparently overlooked in general, that psychogenic pain disorders 'appear to be linked to stressful life events and long-term life problems, indicating the need for a thorough history clinical assessment and the appropriate conservative forms of management'.

The pain patient

The relationship between personality traits, by which one means the unchanging personality of the individual, and the psychological status of patients with chronic orofacial pain is not fully understood. Moulton (1955) and Lupton (1969) described distinct personality types, reviewed by Greene, Olson and Laskin (1982) as:

– 'hypernormals' who were considered dominant, independent, and super efficient;
– 'normals' without emotional problems; and

– 'psychoneurotics' with emotional and personality problems, and often with associated psychophysiological problems of peptic ulcer, colitis, low back pain, hypertension, skin lesions.

However, there is no one discernible personality profile that predisposes to chronic orofacial pain, but rather the presence of a psychological predisposition (Green, Olson and Laskin, 1982) – the so-called 'vulnerable pain person', whose coping skills do not allow them to adequately manage stressful life events. Such individuals tend to fall into three groups:
(a) the psychiatrically normal individual who is subject to stress;
(b) the patient suffering a psychiatric illness such as an anxiety neurosis, depression or psychosis; and
(c) the personality trait where there is an unchanging tendency to somatization or hypochondriasis.

States of anxiety, depression or emotional stress have long been associated with chronic orofacial pain (Moulton, 1955; Lupton, 1969). Greene, Olson and Laskin (1982) recognized the difficulty of identifying whether the pain problem was caused by the psychiatric condition or whether it was caused by the presence of chronic orofacial pain. Malow, Grimm and Olson (1980) in an assessment of anxiety found higher levels of anxiety in patients with myofascial pain dysfunction when compared with asymptomatic controls, but the differences were not statistically significant. It is apparent, however, that anxiety levels are raised by the presence of chronic orofacial pain.

Feinmann and Harris (1984) found that 55% of their pain patients were psychiatrically normal; of the remainder, many of the 20% with an identifiable depressive illness lost their depression with reassurance and medication before their pain. This suggested that the depression resulted from the pain. However, most patients had adverse life events (bereavement, marital disharmony, work problems, alcoholism) usually within six months prior to the onset of pain.

2.3.2 Clinical features

The identification of a pain of psychogenic origin may only be made if there is no known physical cause or pathophysiological mechanism to account for the painful condition, and there is evidence of the presence of contributing psychological factors (Dworkin and Burgess, 1987).

The classification in Table 2.5 is based on studies by Feinmann and Harris (1984a,b), and reviews by Rees and Harris (1978), Scott and Humphreys (1987) and Dworkin and Burgess (1987). However, in this chapter jaw muscle and TM joint pain are described separately to emphasize the dental management.

Pain of psychogenic origin presents with the following general features:

– the location does not follow the anatomical distribution of the nerves;
– it may occur bilaterally;
– it is often continuous with little fluctuation in intensity;
– it generally does not awaken the patient from sleep;

– previous treatment may be successful but relapse after cessation of treatment is common; and
– the patient may link the pain with emotional stress, and may break down in the reporting of these circumstances.

Whatever the features that are suggestive of psychogenic pain, a possible organic cause must be fully investigated in each situation.

Pain of psychogenic origin is thought to arise in three ways:

1. Muscle or vascular tension which is common in neurotic disorders of anxiety, depression or hypochondriasis;
2. Hallucination may accompany psychotic disorders of schizophrenia or endogenous depression;
3. Conversion hysteria may arise by repressed emotional conflict which is converted to peripheral somatic symptoms.

Feinmann and Harris (1984a,b) classify psychogenic orofacial pain into four categories:

1. Facial arthromyalgia which includes TM joint and myofascial pain dysfunction syndrome;
2. Atypical facial pain (idiopathic facial pain);
3. Atypical odontalgia (phantom tooth pain);
4. Oral dysaesthesia, which includes altered sensations of tongue – glossodynia (painful tongue) and glossopyrosis (burning tongue). This term also includes burning or altered sensations of lips, gingival or denture-bearing areas, in the absence of an obvious physical cause. These would include a poorly fitting denture base, gingival irritation from a partial denture retainer or denture base, newly-fitted complete dentures where anterior tooth position is too far labial or grossly over-contoured flanges which may irritate lips.

Many patients suffer these pains sequentially or simultaneously together with headache, neck and back pain, dermatitis, pruritus and irritable colon.

Table 2.5 categorizes craniomandibular pain of psychogenic origin with suggested pathophysiological and psychological mechanisms.

(a) TM joint dysfunction

TM joint dysfunction and myofascial pain dysfunction syndrome are described separately in this chapter (see Sections 2.4 and 2.5) so that specific dental procedures that this author considers important for dental clinicians to understand may be described. It is emphasized that cases refractory to such management should be treated medically.

(b) Phantom tooth pain

Phantom tooth pain or atypical odontalgia is discussed elsewhere in this chapter (see Section 2.2.3).

(c) Atypical facial pain

Atypical facial pain presents with the general features of pain of psychogenic origin, together with the following:

Table 2.5 Craniomandibular pain of psychogenic origin (adapted from Dworkin and Burgess, 1987; Feinmann and Harris, 1984a,b; Scott and Humphreys, 1987)

Type of pain	Pathophysiological mechanism suggested	Physiological mechanism suggested
Myogenous pain and dysfunction	Sustained contraction of jaw muscles	Stress, anxiety, depression, somatization
Tension headache	Sustained contraction of forehead and cervical muscles	Stress, anxiety, depression, somatization
Delusional or hallucinatory disorders – dysmorphophobia	Not known	Profound thought disorder, psychosis
Atypical facial pain. Idiopathic facial pain	Not known	Stress, anxiety, depression, conversion reactions, and hypochondriacal concerns in the absence of a major mental disturbance
Oral dysaesthesia	Not known	
Atypical odontalgia or phantom tooth pain	Not known	

a dull or throbbing ache that is poorly localized and vaguely described. It usually has a non-anatomical distribution, and may be bilateral. There may be associated features of:

sleep disturbance
lethargy
tension
irritability and
agitation.

It is classified by Harris and Feinmann (1984a) as not involving the TM joints or jaw muscles. Scott and Humphreys (1987) include TM joint dysfunction syndrome in this category. This author agrees that chronic intractable pain in the TM joints could be classified as atypical facial pain. However, most TM joint pain problems presenting in clinical practice as specific TM joint problems should be managed by the dental practitioner. Feinmann and Harris (1984a) make this point and add that 10–20% will require supportive psychiatric care.

(d) Hypochondriasis
This has been described by Pilowsky (1978) as a form of abnormal illness behaviour (see Chapter 1, Section 1.1.2). The head and neck are the areas most frequently associated with hypochondriasis, which may have an underlying psychiatric basis such as depression, hysteria, phobic anxiety or personality disorder. Patients present with a variety of clinical signs including:

– pain,
– fear of cancer, and
– a strong belief that they have a specific disease.

This is considered to be a hypochondriacal neurosis where there is sufficient insight to respond to reassurance. If not, the problem is considered to be a hypochondriacal psychosis (see (e)).

They may also reveal general features of depressive illness such as:

– low mood,
– disturbed sleep,
– loss of interest in work, family, pleasure,
– poor concentration,
– loss of energy,
– loss of appetite,
– loss of weight, and
– loss of libido.

(e) Monosymptomatic hypochondriacal psychosis (MHP)

This may present with pain, discomfort or a distortion of taste. It is a chronic delusion with a false but unshakeable belief that is not amenable to reason. If related to a distorted body image (Munro, 1978; Scott and Humphreys, 1987), the condition is called dysmorphophobia or morpho-dysphoria. Here, the preoccupation is with such features as the nose, jaws, teeth crown shape and colour. However, the concern is in excess of the clinical findings which may be normal. Furthermore, all attempts to alter the nose, crowns or bridgework are doomed to failure. The phantom bite (Marbach, Varoscak and Blank, 1983) appears to be a chronic disturbance in proprioception (see Section 2.2.3(e)) with an obsessional psychotic desire to seek correction by repeated dental procedures. Again, such treatment fails and should be avoided. Most psychotic conditions respond well to specific medication – flupenthixol or trifluoperazine, together with frequent firm reassurance (Harris, 1991; personal communication).

It frequently follows irreversible dental procedures and has been reported after occlusal adjustment, fixed restorations and orthodontic treatment. Patients have a common history of multiple dental procedures and often present with a selection of their previous, but unsuccessful, partial or complete dentures, study casts before and after crown procedures, and a collection of radiographs. This is discussed further in Chapter 5 as it relates to occlusal adjustment.

Experiences such as these emphasize the need for careful case selection and treatment planning, the necessity to develop an understanding of one's patient's needs and anxieties, to adopt a conservative approach wherever possible and ensure that the patient is fully informed of the procedures and the reasons for them.

Moulton (1966) made the following suggestions which are of special importance in the management of craniomandibular pain, but are important for all clinical procedures:

1. Develop an atmosphere conducive to rational cooperation from the first appointment;
2. Trust and mutual respect must grow or hostility and misunderstanding will develop;
3. Clinicians' attitude should be of thoughtful, non-judgemental inquiry;

4. Clinicians must be aware of the degree of anxiety of the patient and the possible emotional meaning that the symptoms may have.

2.3.3 Management

Medical management as described by Feinmann and Harris (1984b), Feinmann (1985) and Scott and Humphreys (1987) is the method of choice. The dentist should, as well, seek the support of the patient's physician to assist in the management of chronic conditions; and particularly where medication is to be used, a thorough understanding of their complexity is important and their prescription through medical consultation is essential.

The tricyclic antidepressants appear to have a prophylactic action in aborting many chronic and recurrent pains. Not only are they effective with craniomandibular disorders of psychogenic origin and atypical facial pain, but also with migraine, tension headaches and back aches. Unfortunately, some patients are reluctant to take antidepressant medication unless it is emphasized that it has a marked effect in eliminating pain in non-depressed patients. The neuropharmacological action is unknown, but it is thought to be an enhancement of the natural central amine analgesic effect.

Reassurance consisting of an explanation of the relationship of adverse life events and the onset of pain in blood vessels and muscles is essential. Also, it is essential to indicate that the medication may make the patient a little drowsy on waking, cause a dry mouth and occasionally constipation. All such effects recede with the low dose prescribed.

1. Counselling for a small percentage of disturbed patients is best carried out by a psychologist or psychiatrist, but the sympathetic rapport established by the dentist is also important.
2. Tricyclic antidepressant –
   nortriptyline
   dose: 10–20 mg nocte for 6 weeks
   then 25–50 mg and 100 mg nocte if needed.
3. If there is inadequate response after 2 weeks
   flupenthixol
   dose: 0.5 mg t.d.s.
   or
   a monoamine oxidase inhibitor, Parstelin (trifluoperazine and tranyl-cypromine)
   dose: 1 t.d.s. at 8 am, 12 noon and 4 pm is useful in refractory cases.

The obsessional psychotic hypochondriacal problems tend to respond much better to phenothiazines such as trifluoperazine and flupenthixol (Harris, 1991; personal communication).

2.4 Muscle pain

2.4.1 Introduction

Skeletal muscle through the body may develop pain in a variety of ways, and although jaw muscles have a unique functional importance, there are many similarities between pain developed in the jaw and other muscle systems, such as limb and spinal muscles (Wyke, 1977). The differing aetiology of acute or short-term and chronic or long-term muscle pain will be reviewed in the light of clinical treatment and research data. The possible significance of the occlusion in these mechanisms will be discussed.

Pain from muscle has been described by a variety of terms, and the following are the most commonly applied to pain in jaw muscles:

myalgia (general term for muscle pain) – Harris (1974);
myofascial pain (trigger areas in myofascial structures when activated by pressure, stretch, movement, heat or cold, which evoke pain over specific referral areas) – Travel and Rinzler (1952), Schwartz (1955);
deep vascular pain (associated with muscle blood vessels and mechanical or chemical irritation of the perivascular nociceptive system) – Wyke (1976);
myogenic, myogenous pain (derived from muscle) – Naeije and Hansson (1986).

Myofascial pain has become the most widely accepted term in physical medicine and applies to muscle pain throughout the body (see Travel and Simons, 1983, for review). The term 'myalgia' is used as the general term for muscle pain, but 'myofascial pain' will also be used where trigger areas and referral zones of pain are described. However, irrespective of the term used, the important criteria are the mechanisms and aetiology of the problems presenting for treatment. It is important to distinguish between 'myofascial pain' as a general term for pain arising from skeletal muscle, and 'myofascial pain dysfunction syndrome', as a specific myofascial pain problem with defined clinical features as described by Laskin (1969).

2.4.2 Acute muscle pain

Acute muscle pain may occur as a result of three main factors – mechanical trauma, muscle fatigue and reflex muscle hyperactivity (Table 2.6).

(a) Mechanical trauma

Macrotrauma to muscle may arise from an 'external' source as an external injury – contact sports, blow to face, fall or intra-oral surgery and particularly the surgical removal of an impacted third molar performed under local anaesthesia. In each case, traumatic injury to jaw muscles causes a break in continuity of muscle protein elements and/or connective tissue sheaths with inflammation and alteration in the extracellular fluid. Chemical and mechanical stimulation of the perivascular nerve plexus evokes nociceptive afferents with the development of myalgia (Award, 1973). Table 2.7 lists the chemical products of ischaemia (associated with fatigue) and inflammation (associated with trauma) which stimulate perivascular nerve fibres and generate pain.

Microtrauma implies trauma in the absence of an obvious external force. However, 'internal' forces may also provide microtrauma to muscle protein or connective tissue elements with resulting inflammation, as described above. Common causes are yawning and parafunction,

Table 2.6 Muscle pain – myalgia

TRAUMA

Muscle – inflammation:
  Muscle fibres
  Connective tissue elements

FATIGUE

– Oedema
– Complex – physiology
         – biochemistry
         – psychophysiology
– Blood flow – relative ischaemia
– Sympathetic vasomotor
  responses
– Intramuscular substrate
  transport impaired
– Susceptible individuals

Muscle pain may arise from macro- or microtrauma to muscle and from fatigue. Intramuscular changes associated with trauma result in inflammation. Fatigue and associated oedema is a complex phenomenon.

Table 2.7 Chemical depolarizing agents

IN ISCHAEMIA
  lactic acid   weakest
  potassium ions

IN INFLAMMATION
  Kinins (e.g. bradykinin)
  5-hydroxytryptamine
  prostaglandins
  histamine   strongest

Chemicals released into extra-cellular tissues in association with blood flow reduction and inflammation, which cause depolarization of nociceptive afferents in the region, resulting in pain.

especially nocturnal bruxism during which sustained anterolateral jaw displacement may occur repetitively, leading to muscle fatigue or microtrauma with inflammation and myalgia.

Parafunctional jaw movements are those not related to functions of mastication, swallowing and speech, and include jaw clenching, tooth grinding (which may occur in a forward or lateral direction), tooth tapping, and forced jaw postures in which teeth are interlocked (such as holding the jaw forward in a forced protrusion with the anterior teeth inlocked in a Class III relationship).

The commonest presenting form appears to be lateral parafunction as indicated by wear facets, particularly on anterior teeth. This is likely to be the most destructive of teeth and articular tissues, and may lead to muscle pain.

Sustained jaw muscle contraction is required to maintain the jaw in an eccentric position where the system has reduced resistance to loading, especially in the absence of posterior supporting tooth contacts on working and non-working sides. With centric bruxism, however, where posterior tooth support is present, loading is best resisted by the system.

Parafunction may occur during the day (diurnal) or at night (nocturnal) and it is not uncommon for people to be unaware of either diurnal or nocturnal parafunction.

(b) Muscle fatigue

Jaw muscle fatigue resulting in myalgia and tenderness to palpation may arise as a result of sustained activity. The mechanism responsible for muscle fatigue is complex and not fully understood. An association between fatigue and inadequate blood flow as a result of sustained contraction (Basmajian, 1979) may exist. In such cases, venous drainage from muscle which normally removes accumulated metabolites derived from muscle contraction is unable to do so at the required rate and leads to fatigue and myalgia. This mechanism is, however, much more complex.

Franks (1965a,b) identified the importance of muscle hyperactivity and bruxism as a direct cause of craniomandibular dysfunction. Christensen (1971, 1979) investigated the relationship in healthy subjects between experimental tooth clenching and the resulting muscle fatigue and facial pain. He confirmed that experimental clenching in young healthy adults may induce muscle pain, dull in quality, that is most commonly observed in the temple, cheeks and supraorbital areas, as well as TM joints and the teeth.

Using Xenon-133 clearance to assess blood flow changes in masseter and temporal muscles, Bonde-Petersen and Christensen (1973) found that there is a three-fold increase in blood flow, i.e. hyperaemia, during tooth grinding, but only half this increase in blood flow during tooth clenching for three minutes. This suggests that the resulting facial pain is not due to muscle ischaemia. Studies by Rasmussen *et al.* (1977) and Møller, Rasmussen and Bonde-Petersen (1979) showed that in asymptomatic adults lying supine, clenching for 90 seconds at a bite force greater than 15–20% of maximal clenching, blood flow continued. Clenching was followed by a significant hyperaemia and this response indicates the presence of relative ischaemia in the muscle. They concluded that ischaemia and contraction are inseparable factors in muscle pain, and that tissue displacement in contraction causes compression of larger vessels followed by a marked post-exercise hyperaemia and myalgia.

In a later review of blood flow and mastication, Møller (1985) observed that elevator muscle blood flow increased linearly with intensity of contraction, but during the closing stroke, the elevator activity may cause circulatory arrest, with blood flow returning during the tooth contact phase. Møller proposed firstly that the tooth contact phase is critical for maintaining muscle function and avoiding fatigue; and secondly that muscle strength is an important influencing factor since subjects with weak elevator muscles are more susceptible to contraction overload, and so fatigue and myalgia, than subjects with greater muscle strength.

Montiero (1990) found that ^{133}Xe clearance was not as reliable as laser doppler flowmetry for assessing blood flow and this may explain the apparent disagreement in his results and those obtained from studies by Bonde-Petersen and Christensen (1973).

Furthermore, jaw muscle endurance appears to involve a more complicated mechanism than limb muscle endurance, as exemplified by the following:

1. It appears that studies using visual feedback to maintain bite force are accompanied by rotation of synergistic muscle EMG to minimize the effects of fatigue (Hellsing and Lindström, 1983).
2. Although progressive fatigue and pain are associated with sustained contraction (Christensen, 1979), pain is not the exclusive limiting factor. Naeije and Zorn (1981) found that some subjects stopped clenching because of local fatigue in the absence of pain. It appears that in contrast with limb muscles, affective and motivational factors are involved, i.e. jaw clenching is a complex psycho-physiological activity (Montiero, 1990).

   Also, patients with CMDs show postural EMG activity in anterior and posterior temporal and masseter muscles that is twice that of the asymptomatic controls (Sheikholeslam, Møller and Lous, 1982).

   Both these features suggest that there may be a specific group of susceptible patients who suffer with CMDs.
3. During moderate isometric contraction (above 25% maximum voluntary contraction) there is a rapid decrease in endurance, masseter discomfort, fatigue and pain. This is thought to be due to local fatigue from relative ischaemia (as the response occurs before depletion of muscle substrate).

   There is considerable blood flow at the beginning and end of each chewing cycle; however, it appears that blood flow continues at most levels of activity in the chewing cycle (Montiero, 1990).
4. During low levels of contraction, blood flow appears to be adequate in masseter to satisfy demands. Thus the muscle pain reported by patients appears to be unrelated to the relative ischaemia.
5. Local fatigue without pain causes some subjects to stop clenching, even though blood flow changes were similar in all subjects (Montiero,

1990). Thus, blood flow responses are unrelated to pain, although they are in all instances elicited by reflex responses of sympathetic vasomotor fibres (and possibly other responses) in A-delta and C-fibres (McCloskey and Mitchell, 1972).

6. Sjögaard, Savard and Juel (1988) have suggested a mechanism for muscle fatigue, independent of relative ischaemia. Fatigue is due to:
(a) increased muscle membrane permeability;
(b) passage of intracellular fluid into the interstitial space;
(c) development of oedema; and
(d) impairment of substrate transport within the muscle.

Oedema was described by Christensen (1970) after experimental clenching in asymptomatic subjects, and it is observed in patients with CMDs.

In summary, it appears that sustained jaw muscle contraction leads to varying degrees of relative ischaemia, i.e. in certain regions of the muscle, and is followed by post-contraction hyperaemia. However, blood flow continues at varying levels throughout the chewing cycle. Muscle pain may be experienced but fatigue may occur without pain. Blood flow changes are related to reflex sympathetic vasomotor responses and a change in muscle fibre membrane permeability that results in local muscle oedema. Apart from the identified physiological responses there may be other physiological and biological changes, as yet unknown. As well, jaw muscle fatigue may have a psychological component, and its occurrence may predominate in a specific group of susceptible individuals.

(c) Reflex muscle hyperactivity
The arrangement of the teeth has a direct influence on jaw muscle coordination.

Muscle activity is controlled by a variable balance of peripheral and central nervous system influences (see Klineberg, 1991, Chapter 2). Peripheral influences are both neurological and physical. Neurological influences include feedback from mechanoreceptors in orofacial tissues, such as skin, oral mucosa, periosteum, periodontium and jaw muscles. They provide afferent influences to jaw muscle motoneurones that may, when circumstances require, allow appropriate changes in coordinated muscle activity and jaw displacement to control velocity and direction of movement and bite force.

Physical influences are associated with tooth shape and arrangement. They provide directional influences for jaw muscles which are accommodated by appropriate neuromuscular coordination.

The hypothesis that alteration in tooth contact pattern, as a result of orthodontic tooth movement, restorative or prosthodontic procedures, tooth loss or other dental treatment may lead to hyperactivity of jaw muscle (or regions within them), spasm and pain, is not supported by critical analysis and current research (Lund and Widmer, 1989).

The possibility that teeth might act as a trigger (via contact interferences) to the development of muscle spasm and pain arose from early studies, such as those by Moyers (1956), Travel (1960) and Ramfjord

(1961). These studies provided a new dimension to dental care and inevitably focused on the teeth and their influences. This information provided a rationale for dental treatment involving alterations in tooth form, height and inter-arch relationships.

The extent to which a less than optimum tooth arrangement affects function is not clear, or even what the terms 'optimum' (good) or 'less than optimum' (poor) means in relation to the jaw muscle system. What is clear, however, is that there is a broad range of tooth sizes, shapes and arrangements occurring in asymptomatic healthy individuals with apparently optimal function that do not require treatment. Many other factors must play a role in defining 'optimum', including skeletal form, jaw arrangement and associated muscle fibre orientation and characteristics. Recent studies of shortened dental arches for instance (Witter, van Elteren and Käyser, 1988; Witter *et al.*, 1990) have found no association between absence of molar teeth and CMDs. Also, it should be recalled that Posselt (1962) originally described a slide from RP to IP in 90% of individuals examined. As this difference in IP and RP is a feature of most dentitions, it would be highly unlikely that its presence would have any relationship with orofacial pain or dysfunction.

Occlusal stability, i.e. the presence of bilateral tooth contacts at IP, during chewing, has an important influence on muscle coordination. Bakke, Møller and Thorsen (1982) showed that activity of contralateral anterior temporal and ipsilateral and contralateral masseter muscles was positively correlated with occlusal stability. During mastication, the strength of muscle contraction increases with bilateral stability at IP, so that tooth arrangements that lead to an unstable IP will affect muscle strength, contraction time and postural activity.

Where posterior teeth have been lost beyond the equilibrium point (as described by Tradowsky and Dworkin (1982) to be in the region of the second bicuspid and first molar), alteration in muscle activity may occur in an attempt to maximize available tooth contact. This will help to reduce the loading at the TM joints during function but may lead to posturing of the jaw in a forward position.

However, drawing an association between such changes in jaw muscle activity and associated orofacial pain is not supported by a current understanding of muscle physiology or clinical studies of muscle activity:

1. Jaw muscles contain a variable proportion of slow, fast and intermediate muscle fibres of varying biochemical and histochemical characteristics and fatigue resistance (Eriksson and Thornell, 1983).
2. The arrangement of motor units in muscle provides the basis on which selective recruitment of motor units is possible, allowing fine adjustment and control of jaw movement (Stålberg and Eriksson, 1987; Lund and Widmer, 1989).
3. There is great variation in jaw movement as described in studies of healthy asymptomatic individuals (Mongini, Tempia-Valenta and Benvegnu, 1986; Pröschel and Hofmann, 1988; Feine, Hutchins and Lund, 1988; Ellis *et al.*, 1990; Mohl *et al.*, 1990), indicating that the associated jaw muscle activity must also be highly variable. It is thus not

possible to attribute symptoms of orofacial pain to variations in jaw displacement or EMG activity without additional data, particularly on the range of activity that exists in healthy, asymptomatic adults. Also, it is important to acknowledge that there are differences associated with:
(a) Age – EMG activity is reduced as age increases (Visser and De Rijke, 1974; Lund and Widmer, 1989);
(b) Sex – muscle activity in women has been reported to be greater than in men performing the same task (Visser and De Rijke, 1974; Lund and Widmer, 1989); and
(c) Facial morphology – jaw size, shape, spatial arrangement (prognathic, retrognathic) must have an influence on muscle mass, fibre orientation, resolution of muscle forces and recorded EMG.

Such factors must be considered when attributing symptoms to changes in muscle activity. To date, no clearly defined description of what is 'normal' has been identified (Lund and Widmer, 1989) although studies in progress are attempting to assess this matter (Howell and Klineberg, unpublished data).

(d) Clinical signs
A number of clinical signs strongly suggest a muscle basis and bruxism either as a primary cause or an associated feature of myalgia:

– Jaw stiffness on awakening (identified by Franks, 1965b). This may prevent further damage or more pain in the affected tissues, e.g. TM joint, muscle, teeth, soft tissues;
– Limited jaw opening on awakening. This may be associated with a jaw muscle protective role and/or interarticular disc displacement. When of muscle origin, the mobility usually increases with jaw stretching after awakening.
– Mucosal ridging was first described by Franks (1965b) on the cheek and/or tongue, indicating sustained pressure of tongue and cheeks against the teeth, associated with repetitive forceful muscle activity.
– The teeth may ache on awakening.
– There may be jaw muscle pain and/or pain referred to the face and neck.

2.4.3 Chronic muscle pain

(a) General features
Not all pain from jaw muscle is of short duration and with an apparent causative mechanism. Where pain has been present for months or years, the initial aetiological factor becomes obscured and is no longer relevant to the now more complex chronic pain problem.

Chronic muscle pain may have a psychogenic basis and occurs in the head and face either as:
pain in jaw muscles, or
muscle contraction or tension headache.

The mechanism is thought to be due to prolonged muscle contraction and muscle fatigue, but this is not proven.

The aetiology is associated with:
stress, anxiety, depression and
sometimes irritability and anger (Dworkin and Burgess, 1987).

Pain of this type in jaw muscles has many features in common with chronic skeletal muscle pain in other parts of the body, e.g. tension headache and low back pain (Sternbach, 1974).

However, it is important to emphasize that most pain patients that present to Pain Clinics have an organic basis for their pain problem. At Orofacial Pain Clinics in Australia (Reade, Burrows and Gerschman, 1977) and the USA (Marbach, personal communication, 1980), only 2% and 3+% respectively, of patients presented without evidence of an organic basis for the disease, indicating a psychiatric problem. Such a conclusion can only be reached through additional specialist advice, and the conditions cannot be treated with conventional dental therapy, but require a multidisciplinary approach including psychotherapy.

It has been shown experimentally (Yemm, 1971) that physical stress causes muscle hyperactivity and facial pain in a similar pattern to that which occurs clinically from parafunction. The role of emotional stress in the clinical development of orofacial pain has been clearly revealed (Rugh and Solberg, 1976), as well as the fact that non-dental therapy is equally as effective in treatment as a number of hitherto empirical dental procedures (Greene, Olson and Laskin, 1982; Berry and Harris, 1985). Furthermore the presence of chronic pain (either untreated or unsuccessfully treated) aggravates an anxiety state and thereby compounds the pain problem.

Certain general features of chronic pain are repeated below to emphasize the special nature of chronic pain:

1. Pain is a complex phenomenon since it is largely an emotional or psychological experience and management requires the development of a special understanding between clinician and patient (see Chapter 1).
2. There is a significant number of patients who are more susceptible to pain, the so-called 'vulnerable pain person'.
3. A large percentage of patients (25%, Marbach, 1977; Marbach and Lipton, 1978) report stressful life events as precipitating factors in the onset of chronic pain.
4. Psychosocial variables modify an individual's response to pain experiences.
5. Counselling is an important aspect of management of chronic pain.
6. Specific medication has been found to be beneficial in management and includes tricyclic antidepressants and/or monoamine oxidase inhibitors (Feinmann and Harris, 1984b; Feinmann, 1985). Such medication should only be obtained through medical consultation.

(b) Myofascial pain dysfunction syndrome
Myofascial pain dysfunction or MPD syndrome was introduced by Laskin (1969) to describe a mechanism for pain and dysfunction of the jaw joint and jaw muscle system, based on a psycho-physiological understanding of cause and effect. The most common cause was proposed to be muscle fatigue resulting from chronic oral habits and generated by psychological

stress leading to muscle spasm. It was considered that the cause of 'myospasm' was threefold – muscle overextension, overcontraction and/or fatigue.

Specific clinical features were described as:

1. Pain felt in the ear or pre-auricular area;
2. Jaw muscle tenderness;
3. Clicking or popping sounds in the TM joint;
4. Limited jaw opening and/or deviation of the jaw on opening;
5. Absence of clinical radiographic or biochemical evidence of organic changes in the TM joints;
6. Lack of tenderness of the TM joints when palpated via the external ear.

Associated features noted are:

1. Associated history of migraine, ulcer, dermatitis;
2. Presence of chronic oral habits – clenching or grinding teeth, chewing gum, biting on hard objects;
3. No radiographic evidence of TM joint abnormality;
4. The presence of stress as a significant factor (shown by elevated urine catecholamine levels) suggest that they could be a response to pain.

This theory proposed that changes in the system such as occlusal disharmonies, degenerative arthritis and muscle contracture arose as a result of the condition rather than as a cause. This was a refreshingly modern approach and one that took issue with the commonly held opinion that occlusal discrepancies are a primary cause of orofacial pain. Laskin extended the views of Schwartz (1955), and built on the behavioural studies of Lupton (1969) and the new understanding of orofacial pain and dysfunction that was emerging from studies of human behaviour, emotional stress and anxiety by Goldstein (1964), Moulton (1955, 1966) and others. The theory linked behaviour and muscle symptoms with tooth and TM joint features. MPD syndrome has been studied extensively since that time by Laskin and co-workers and particularly by Greene: Greene and Laskin (1972, 1974), Greene (1973), Goodman, Greene and Laskin (1976), Mercuri, Olson and Laskin (1979), Olson (1980) and Greene, Olson and Laskin (1982).

In a review by Greene, Olson and Laskin (1982) a number of conclusions were made indicating a progressive understanding of the aetiology and clinical signs. They concluded that there is not a particular personality trait or profile that predisposes to MPD, but rather a combination of a predisposition to develop dysfunction, psychological and physical stress and the person's ability to cope with these problems. In relation to psychological circumstances, they concluded that they were uncertain as to whether the stress, anxiety and depression were a cause or an effect, and that chronic symptoms are likely to increase anxiety and that depression was probably a result of concern about health rather than a cause of illness. In relation to stress, they reported that MPD patients showed 'response specificity' – since stress is known to evoke a variety of responses in different individuals (such as headache, duodenal ulcer, colitis, dermatitis or jaw muscle pain) – with a particular response becoming the 'pathologic' or dominant one. The authors also acknowledged that central nervous system hyperactivity (Yemm, 1979) was an important contributing factor.

Dworkin and Burgess (1987) have classified MPD together with muscle tension or contraction headache as a chronic orofacial pain of psychological origin with somatoform features (i.e. involving jaw muscles), the cause being stress, anxiety and depression (see Table 2.5).

2.4.4 Management

(a) General

A number of treatment approaches are possible for acute and chronic pain problems. Acute and chronic pain should be managed differently.

(i) Where a diagnosis of an acute (short duration) pain is made, the treatment options are varied (Table 2.8) but the aim is to alleviate the pain problem as quickly as possible and this approach also implies simple treatment. There may be a need for extensive treatment later, but that should not influence initial therapy.

Table 2.8 Management of muscle pain

	Acute pain	*Chronic pain*
Medication	possibly	essential
Vapo coolant spray	possibly	
Physiotherapy	possibly	
Occlusal splint	yes	possibly
Occlusal adjustment	possibly	not appropriate
Counselling	necessary	essential

(ii) In the case of chronic pain, the management approach should be to confirm a diagnosis and elect simple reversible procedures. MPD syndrome is included in this category of chronic pain. Acute myofascial pain, as defined by Travel (1960), is managed according to the approach for acute pain, whilst MPD syndrome is a different clinical problem.

It has been clearly illustrated (Greene and Laskin, 1972, 1974; Goodman, Greene and Laskin, 1976) that reversible therapy is the most appropriate means of management and these studies confirmed the placebo response to therapy. They also acknowledged that no one treatment is universally appropriate, and that a variety of conservative therapies (such as jaw exercises, occlusal splints, joint and muscle injections, physiotherapy, psychological counselling and medication – analgesics, antidepressants) are effective (Greene and Laskin, 1974).

Specific forms of physical therapy (such as occlusal equilibration, increased vertical dimension of occlusion with fixed prosthodontics and surgery) did not improve the success rate. Greene and Laskin (1974) concluded that failure to respond to treatment is not related to whether the physical therapy was insufficient or incorrect, but rather to complex psychological factors that interfere with the dentist–patient relationship (see Section 2.3).

As a result of these features of chronic pain, it is now widely acknowledged that behavioural approaches to management are essential, that placebo effects, spontaneous remissions and cyclical fluctuations occur, and that no one particular treatment has been shown to be clearly more successful than other methods. A variety of treatment approaches of a reversible nature are recommended (Zarb and Speck, 1977; Greene and Laskin, 1982; Griffiths, 1983; Mejersjö and Carlsson, 1983; Feinmann and Harris, 1984a,b; Wedel and Carlsson, 1985; Scott and Humphreys, 1987).

(iii) It is important to note that certain psychosocial influences appear to be present in the case of patients who seek treatment for their facial pain problem (Marbach and Lipton, 1978), since epidemiological studies (Helkimo, 1976), have shown that a far greater percentage of people have pain and other symptoms of myofascial pain dysfunction, but do not seek treatment.

Alternatively, the problem of chronicity may to some extent be engendered in the health care system itself: firstly because of the ever-present problem of too little time available for adequate consultation and therapy; secondly, general clinicians and specialists in medicine and dentistry inevitably consider pain problems within the framework of their own disciplines, and therefore the first person to offer and administer definitive treatment plays a critical role in the management of myofascial pain dysfunction. Unfortunately a simplistic approach is likely to be unsuccessful because of the psychogenic features of facial pain.

If initial therapy does not bring about relief of symptoms, then the next clinician to offer treatment begins at a disadvantage. The clinician must establish a rapport with the patient to gain their confidence and devote adequate consultation time to allow an accurate diagnosis to be made. Treatment may then begin with a good prognosis. In this way, unnecessary and destructive treatments such as tooth extractions, removal and replacement of restorations, fitting of crowns, root canal therapies, extensive prosthodontic procedures or repeated occlusal adjustments may be avoided. Successive treatments that do not provide any beneficial effect for the patient compound the problem, and psychological disorders of depression, anxiety, hysteria and hypochondriasis may develop, because of the apparently helpless situation in which patients find themselves.

(iv) A diagnosis of muscle involvement may be made on the basis of:
- the known referral patterns from jaw and cervical muscles to superficial tissues of head and neck (Figure 2.1);
- palpation tenderness of individual jaw and cervical muscles (Figure 2.2); and
- provocation tests (Krogh-Poulsen and Olsson, 1969) designed to provoke jaw muscle pain in susceptible muscles. This routinely involves matching bruxofacets on opposing teeth and having the patient clench in that jaw position for one half to one minute. The development of discomfort and/or pain confirms jaw clenching in that way to be a cause of muscle pain.

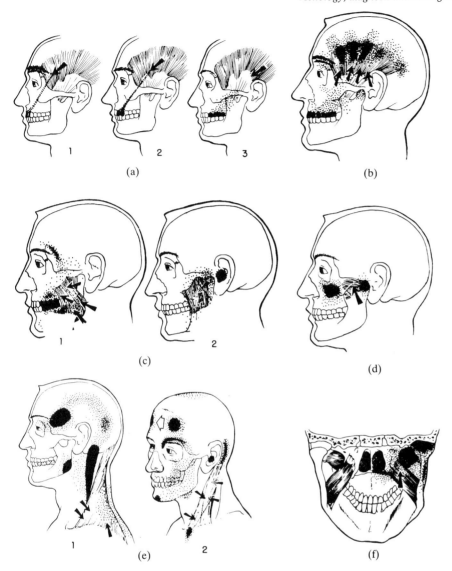

Figure 2.1 Pain referral zones from jaw and cervical muscles (From Travel, 1960 with permission)

(a) Pain referral sites from three regions of temporal muscle. Note referral to maxillary incisor teeth, and to eyebrow area (1) from anterior temporal fibres; to canine and bicuspid teeth from middle temporal area (2); and to molar teeth from posterior fibres (3).

(b) Pain referral pattern from all areas of temporal muscle when the whole muscle is involved. Note that pain is felt in the muscle, and referred to maxillary teeth and eyebrow areas.

(c) Pain referral pattern from superficial masseter (1). Note referral to posterior teeth, temple area and jaw. Pain referral from deep masseter (2) to pre-auricular area and ear.

(d) Pain referral pattern from lateral pterygoid. Note referral to region of root of zygoma and to TM joint. This is the most common means of pain referral to the TM joint.

(e) Pain referral pattern from trapezius (1). Note referral to side of neck, angle of mandible and temple area. Pain referral pattern from sternomastoid (2). Note referral to sternum, ear, postauricular area, chin, temple and eyebrow area.

(f) Pain referral pattern from medial pterygoid to deep structures – palate, maxilla, TM joint.

(b) Clinical approach

(i) Vapo-coolant*/local anaesthesia The diagnostic value of a vapo-coolant (e.g. ethylchloride spray) (Travel, 1960; Kraus, 1969; Solberg, 1979; Travel and Simons, 1983) for superficial muscles, and local anaesthetic infiltration for superficial and deep muscles may be required if there is still uncertainty about the involvement of particular muscles.

---

*Bengué; Ethylchloride; Bengué & Co. Ltd, Maidenhead, Berks SL6 1RD, UK;
PR Spray (dichlorodifluoromethane 15% + trichlorofluoromethane 85%); The Boots Company PLC, Nottingham, Notts NG2 3AA, UK;
Skefron (dichlorodifluoromethane 15% + trichlorofluoromethane 15%); Smith Kline & French Laboratories, Mundells, Welwyn Garden City, Herts AL7 1EY, UK;
Frezan (dichlorotetrafluoroethane 65% + ethylchloride 15.5%); Drug Houses of Australia, Turella 2205, Australia.

These two techniques are primarily of diagnostic value, but the analgesic effects may long outlast the period of anaesthesia. It is proposed that this occurs because the anaesthesia of superficial tissues varies the afferent input to the brainstem and alters the inhibitory balance of transmission neurones in the nucleus caudalis of the spinal tract of the trigeminal system (see Chapter 1, Section 1.1.3 and Figure 1.4); once the anaesthetic effects have worn off, a changed inhibitory balance has developed which may remain for an extended time, and in this way maintains analgesia.

(ii) Medication A variety of medications may be suitable for acute muscle pain: analgesics provide symptomatic relief for the pain (Table 2.9);

Table 2.9 Analgesics

Active ingredient	Proprietary name	Manufacturer
Aspirin (900 mg)	Disprin (300 mg) Sig. 3 tabs 4 hourly p.r.n.	Reckitt & Colman
Dextropropoxyphene HCL (32.5 mg) + Paracetamol (32.5 mg)	Digesic Sig. 2 tabs 4 hourly p.r.n.	Dista
Paracetamol (1 g)	Panadol Sig. 2 tabs 4 hourly p.r.n.	Winthrop

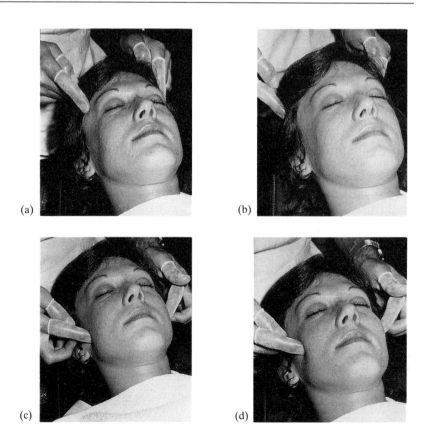

(a)

(b)

(c)

(d)

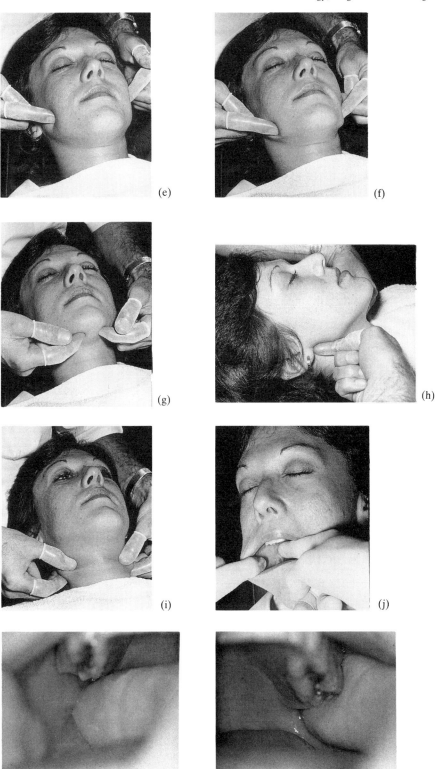

Figure 2.2 Jaw muscle palpation.
A. Superficial muscles: (a)
anterior temporalis m; (b) Middle-
posterior temporalis m; (c) Deep
masseter m; (d) Superficial
masseter m – origin; (e) Superficial
masseter m – body; (f) Superficial
masseter m – insertion;
(g) Anterior digastric m;
(h) Posterior digastric m;
(i) Sternomastoid m – body.
   B. Intra-oral palpation:
(j) Temporal tendon; (k) Medial
pterygoid; (l) Lateral pterygoid

Table 2.10 Muscle relaxants

Active ingredient	Proprietary name	Manufacturer
Diazepam	Ducene (2, 5 mg) Sig. 2 mg t.i.d.	Sauter
	Pro-Pam (2, 5, 10 mg) Sig. 2 mg t.i.d.	Protea
	Valium (2, 5, 10 mg) Sig. 2 mg t.i.d.	Roche
Orphenadrine citrate	Norflex (100 mg) Sig. 100 mg b.d.	Riker
	Norgesic (35 mg with paracetamol 450 mg) Sig. 2 tabs t.i.d.	Riker
Methocarbamol	Robaxin (500 mg) Sig. 3 tabs q.i.d. for 2–3 days	A. H. Robins

Table 2.11 Antidepressants

Active ingredient	Proprietary name	Manufacturer
Amytriptyline hydrochloride	Tryptanol (10, 25, 50 mg) Sig. 50–100 mg daily	Frost
	Saroten (25 mg) Sig. 25 mg t.i.d.	Nicholas
	Laroxyl (10, 25 mg) Sig. 25 mg b.d.	Roche
	Amitrip (25 mg) Sig. 25 mg t.i.d. to a max. of 150 mg daily	Protea
Nortriptyline	Allegron (10, 25 mg) Sig. 75–100 mg daily in divided doses	Dista
	Nortab (10, 25 mg) Sig. 25 mg t.i.d.	Squibb
Dothiepin hydrochloride	Prothiaden (25, 75 mg) Sig. 25 mg t.i.d. increasing to a max. of 200 mg daily	Boots
Phenelzine	Nardil (15 mg) Sig. 15 mg t.i.d.	Warner
Imipramine HCl	Imiprin (10, 25 mg) Sig. 25 mg t.i.d.	Protea
	Tofranil (10, 25 mg) Sig. 25 mg t.i.d.	Geigy
Tranylcypromine sulphate	Parnate (10 mg) Sig. 10 mg b.d.	Smith, Kline & French
	Parstelin (10 mg) Sig. 10 mg b.d.	Smith, Kline & French

sedatives for muscle relaxation are valuable where muscle hyperactivity and stress induced parafunction are present (Table 2.10); Chronic myofascial pain may require antidepressant drug therapy over a period of 6 to 12 weeks (Table 2.11), and this may be supplemented by small doses of a phenothiazine drug. The medication is used independently of its antidepressant effect. Feinmann and Harris (1984a,b) recommend antidepressant nortriptyline, 10–100 mg (av. 50 mg) nocte, and supplemented by the antipsychotic drug Stelazine (trifluoperazine), 2–4 mg (2–4 tabs) each morning. Prescription of psychotropic drugs through medical consultation must be emphasized.

(iii) Physiotherapy Table 2.12 lists commonly employed physiotherapy procedures some of which are appropriate for jaw muscle and jaw joint dysfunction. Those procedures appropriate for jaw muscle dysfunction are indicated below.

1. Moist heat has a soothing effect as well as increasing vascularity to aid the resolution of inflammation.
2. Stretch–relax exercises are particularly valuable for muscle dysfunction, and are effective in breaking down muscle adhesions thereby increasing the range of joint mobility. This, maybe, also effective in breaking down intra-articular adhesions.
3. Heat and ultrasound: Where sudden trauma rapidly and forcefully translates the condyles, pain may result within 3–6 weeks. This situation may arise following whiplash injuries to the cervical spine which hypertranslates the condyle, or in contact sport injuries. The sudden and extreme jaw and condyle movement may cause trauma to fibres of the superior head of the lateral pterygoid muscle, interarticular disc, synovial linings of anterior joint compartments and posterior attachment tissues.

   Heat applied to the joint area in such cases gives temporary relief. Greater relief may be produced by heat followed by ultrasound therapy (Mahan, 1975) using mechanical vibration of specific configuration with the following prescription (Harris, 1991; personal communication):
   wattage: 1.0 watts/cm^2
   frequency: 3 MHz
   pulse: 1 in 4
   duration: 10 min.
   Lehmann *et al.* (1968) has described that ultrasound will:
   (a) increase the temperature at tissue interfaces deep in the tissues;
   (b) encourage resolution of fibrosis;
   (c) increase the flexibility of connective tissues; and
   (d) stimulate protein synthesis.
   It has been shown also to relieve pain generated by neuromas following peripheral nerve injury.
   The technique requires that:
   (a) Heat be applied to the affected side for a period of 10 min;
   (b) Ultrasound be applied for 5 to 10 min, increasing from 0.5 to 1.1 watts/cm^2 as is tolerated by the patient;

Table 2.12 Physiotherapy

HEAT
– Conduction: moist heat
– Conversion: short wave diathermy, ultrasound

EXERCISES
– Mobilization exercises (stretch:relax)
– Isokinetic or resistance exercises
– Movement awareness exercises

MUSCLE STIMULATION

TRACTION

A number of procedures may be of benefit in the interdisciplinary management of craniomandibular disorders. Some of the procedures indicated may be carried out by the dentist, but referral to a physiotherapist is recommended.

(c) This procedure be repeated during ten treatment sessions over a period of two weeks.

4. Short wave diathermy: This involves the use of a diathermy machine to generate high frequency radio waves that promote temperature increases. The effects produced include:
(a) increase in vascularity of deep tissues;
(b) aiding resolution of inflammation of joint capsules, ligaments and tendons.

(iv) Splint therapy (see Chapter 4)

Muscle pain

All teeth are discluded by the interposition of a carefully designed heat-processed acrylic resin splint that provides flat-plane contact against opposing teeth. A maxillary or mandibular splint may be used depending on the jaw and tooth arrangement, but in most instances a maxillary splint is more appropriate, as it can more readily satisfy design requirements (see Chapter 4).

Such an appliance will allow the jaw to establish an anteroposterior and lateral orientation in the absence of cuspal guidance so that any jaw muscle dysfunction (sustained activity, fatigue, etc.), either generated or enhanced by tooth contact interferences, may resolve. It is 'open-ended' treatment that allows adjustment and modification.

Splint adjustment must continue until a stable jaw position is established. However, if there is no relief within 2–4 weeks following careful initial fitting and adjustments, then this type of therapy is unlikely to provide pain relief. The critical aspect of occlusal splint adjustment is to ensure by the careful use of ultra-fine occlusal tapes* that there is a bilateral distribution of tooth contacts at a guided terminal hinge axis (THA) jaw position, and an absence of posterior supracontacts in lateral or protrusive jaw movements.

Jaw muscle parafunction

Where parafunction involves tooth grinding or jaw clenching, long-term splint therapy prevents continual tooth surface loss as a result of the parafunctional habit. The splint is worn at night and as well during the day when required, particularly during periods of stress and anxiety. Jaw clenching and tooth grinding parafunctions have a psycho-physiological mechanism and have been described as manifestations of daytime stress and anxiety (Solberg, Clark and Rugh, 1975; Ayer, 1979) and are not evoked by tooth contact interferences. Other treatments such as relaxation therapy, biofeedback, hypnosis and massed practice therapy may also be effective (Bailey and Rugh, 1979).

(v) Biofeedback Humans and animals, when provided with new information in the form of biofeedback of internal responses (heart rate,

---

*GHM Foil, Gebr. Hanel-Medizinal, D7440 Nürtingen, Germany.

respiration rate, etc.) and incentives (or rewards) for changing the response, are able to learn to alter a variety of physiological activities voluntarily. This self-regulatory technique has been widely used since the 1970s in clinical treatment and research (Schwartz, 1975).

The capacity of the human brain to regulate dynamic patterns of neural, skeletal and visceral responses arises because of its extraordinary capacity for response specificity. Basmajian (1972) showed that biofeedback applied to voluntary control of skeletal muscle allowed initial control of muscle groups, and with further training allowed control of individual motor unit groups within muscles.

Electromyographic biofeedback is the instantaneous feedback to a patient of muscle tension levels, as measured by the electrical activity of a contracting muscle and feedback by visual, auditory, or other means (Peck and Kraft, 1977). Although EMG monitoring of facial muscle tension has traditionally involved the frontalis muscle, recording from specific muscles for example facial expression (Schwartz, 1975), jaw muscle pain (Clarke and Kardachi, 1977) or back and shoulder pain (Peck and Kraft, 1977) is more accurate and appropriate.

Peck and Kraft (1977) studied the use of biofeedback on tension headache, back and jaw pain. Tension headache and jaw pain patients responded best to EMG biofeedback training. Treatment sessions were twice weekly for half an hour. Surface electrodes were applied to the skin surface overlying key muscles, and visual feedback of the EMG signal monitored the response pattern. Most patients showed a progressive improvement, some more marked than others.

Clarke and Kardachi (1977) and Kardachi and Clarke (1977) applied EMG biofeedback monitoring of affected superficial jaw muscles with auditory feedback during sleep. This alternative approach confirmed the value of EMG biofeedback in management of MPD and bruxism, respectively.

In each case, surface electrodes were placed on the masseter and temporal muscles on the affected side and retained during a full night's sleep. The EMG signal was fed to an earpiece indicating to the subject the level of jaw muscle activity. However, the threshold was adjusted such that only parafunctional or bruxing activity was sampled, the level of signal reflecting the degree of muscle activity. Regular jaw movement activity, such as that accompanying swallowing, was not monitored as the motor unit activity was too low. In this way the subject was alerted to excessive muscle activity during sleep.

The results of these studies of nocturnal EMG biofeedback indicated a marked reduction in facial pain and jaw muscle parafunctional activity.

The results described in these studies reflect the value of EMG biofeedback in the management of clinical pain problems that are directly associated with elevated muscle tension levels. The response of patients to this type of therapy is variable. Individuals differ in their response pattern to stress and similarly to biofeedback therapy. However, studies such as these indicate that the reduction in muscle tension headache using EMG biofeedback training is not a placebo response, but an actual reduction in motor unit activity or muscle tension.

Such management programmes are desirable therapeutic tools to encourage behavioural modification with patient cooperation and involvement. The latter is the key to the success of such treatments long term, since a continuation of the particular relaxation programme is necessary after the period of active treatment, in order to maintain maximum benefit of treatment.

(vi) Stabilization – occlusal adjustment (see Chapter 5) Occlusal adjustment may be desirable in cases of chronic muscle pain, once it has become apparent that splint therapy has been beneficial in relieving pain symptoms. In treatment of chronic pain, splint therapy is an essential prerequisite. Occlusal adjustment is totally inappropriate in cases where splint therapy has not induced relief of symptoms.

Wenneberg, Nystrom and Carlsson (1988) compared the effectiveness of occlusal adjustment and occlusal splint together with jaw exercises and counselling therapies in thirty patients with CMDs. Fifteen patients were in each group. The splint therapy group resulted in 90% improvement, whilst the occlusal adjustment group resulted in 50–60% improvement. The occlusal adjustment group also reported improved occlusal function and a reduction of TM joint sounds. The reasons for the subjective improvement in comfort of the occlusion after occlusal adjustment is discussed in Chapter 5, Section 5.2.3.

It is clear from this study that splint therapy should precede any occlusal adjustment in management of CMDs in order to maximize the effectiveness of this treatment.

During functional jaw movement following occlusal adjustment, the guiding inclines of the teeth now provide an increased functional angle of occlusion. Also, simultaneous contacts on the maximum number of teeth occur at the apex of the functional angle, providing bilaterally balanced jaw support. Møller (1985) has indicated that this is an important feature of occlusal therapy, since relief of jaw muscle dysfunction is dependent upon the development of bilaterally balanced tooth contacts in function, and freedom to perform smooth eccentric jaw movements into and from intercuspal position.

Studies in progress investigating functional jaw movements confirm the need for stable posterior tooth contacts at IP to provide a stable end point for jaw closing. This provides a regular reference point for the commencement of jaw opening which may be important to reset muscle controls (see Section 2.4.2(c) in this Chapter). This also allows regularity of tooth contact and an appropriate pause in elevator muscle contraction. Also, anterior tooth arrangement and contour must allow the jaw to translate anterior to IP as required during early opening or late closing. This requires a certain amount of anteroposterior and lateral freedom at tooth contact.

Figure 2.3 illustrates these features with frontal and sagittal plane tracings of unrestricted jaw movement during chewing. Such tracings in the frontal plane reveal the required precision of jaw movement with a clearly defined apex of the functional angle of occlusion; whilst tracings in the

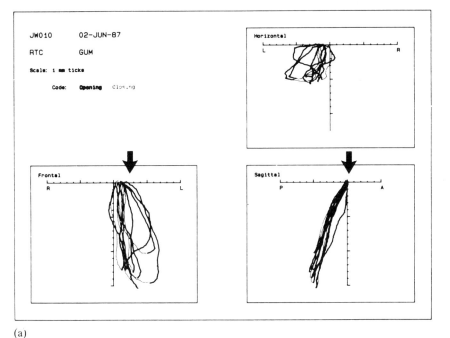

(a)

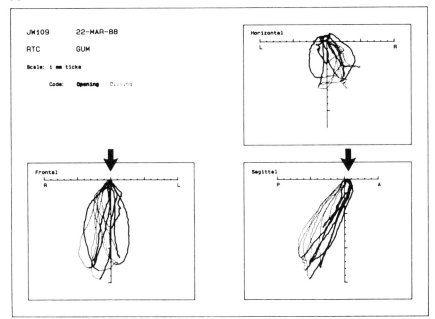

(b)

Figure 2.3 Recordings of jaw movements have been obtained with a Sirognathograph (Siemens AG, Benshein, West Germany) from a patient (♀, 33 years, Class II skeletal and deep overbite) with TM joint dysfunction, during right-sided gum chewing. Two series of composite envelopes of function in three planes are shown, the first was recorded before treatment (2.6.87) and the second after treatment for dysfunction (22.3.88).

(a) Pre-treatment recordings, 2.6.87. The frontal plane recording shows a variable end point for each chewing cycle at IP (arrows). This lack of precision at IP is associated with the presence of TM joint dysfunction. The sagittal plane recording shows a narrow functional angle of occlusion (FAO – author's term) anteroposteriorly as a feature of the deep overbite (arrow). The horizontal plane recording as well as the frontal recording confirm that the patient did not chew on the right as had been requested (RTC).

(b) Post-treatment recordings, 22.3.88. The frontal plane recording shows a well-defined functional angle of occlusion at the end point of each chewing cycle at IP (arrow). This precision of movement is considered to be indicative of a return to asymptomatic function (unpublished data). The sagittal plane recording shows a broader anteroposterior movement, i.e. a broader FAO with some jaw closing movements passing anterior to the starting point at IP (arrow). This 'freedom' in centric, i.e. anteroposterior 'freedom', is considered to be an important feature of optimum anterior guidance and asymptomatic function. The horizontal plane recording confirms the anteroposterior 'freedom', with tracings seen to be forward of the starting point. It also indicates, together with frontal tracings, that the patient is more able to follow the instruction for right side chewing (RTC)

sagittal plane reveal the anteroposterior freedom needed to provide for the anterior component of jaw movement.

These physiological studies allow an objective means of assessment of the occlusal scheme, with particular emphasis on bilateral stability at IP and correctly designed lateral guidance.

2.5 Temporomandibular joint pain

2.5.1 Introduction

Functional disturbances of the TM joints comprise an important component of CMDs and may present clinically as a separate disorder, or may occur in combination with jaw muscle pain (see Section 2.4) and/or craniocervical dysfunctions. All synovial joints are richly innervated, and the presence of a joint dysfunction may reflexly alter jaw muscle activity and in this way may be a cause of jaw muscle hyperactivity and subsequent myalgia.

(a) Craniocervical aspects
Hellsing (1987) and Hellsing *et al.* (1987) examined craniofacial morphology in relation to head and body posture in children and found that the curvature of the lumbar and thoracic spine increased with age and cervical lordosis was directly associated with head posture and mode of breathing (via mouth or nose). The latter influenced resting lip pressure which may influence anterior tooth arrangement. They also found that there was a marked change in EMG activity with changes in head posture:

(i) Flexion (head forward) resulted in:

Posterior cervical muscles – increased EMG
Sternocleidomastoid muscles – unchanged
Infrahyoid muscles – increased EMG
Masseter muscles – unchanged

(ii) Extension (head backward) resulted in:

Posterior cervical muscles – reduced EMG
Sternocleidomastoid muscles – increased EMG
Infrahyoid muscles – increased EMG
Masseter muscles – increased EMG

The increased activity of infrahyoid muscles is probably to maintain hyoid bone orientation and ensure a patent airway.

Such changes in craniocervical posture and jaw and cervical muscle activity, if sustained, could influence craniofacial morphology during growth and development (Fosberg *et al.*, 1985).

It can be seen that craniocervical posture has a close association with jaw posture. The neurological importance of the nucleus caudalis of the spinal nucleus of the trigeminal nerve as a relay centre for cervical and jaw muscle motor control has been described by a number of authors. Abrahams and Richmond (1977) describe the cervical spinal cord and its associations with the trigeminal system as a special receptor system and it is known clinically that damage to neck structures (often as whiplash) causes a variety of symptoms including disturbances of gait, vision and dizziness. A syndrome termed 'cervical ataxia' has been given to this complex of symptoms following injury to the cervical spine. The interrelationship of neck muscle function to the whole well-being of the head is emphasized by these associations.

Abrahams (1977) describes a major role for the trigeminal system in motor control of cervical muscles and the control of head movement. This is in addition to its other major role in nociceptive transmission from orofacial tissues. Cervical nerves C1 to C4 are primarily associated with head posture (Bogduk, 1982) and afferent fibres from C1 to C4 relay in the brainstem to nucleus caudalis of the trigeminal system, the most caudal section of the sensory nucleus of the trigeminal system that relays nociception. Non-nociceptive projections may relay in deeper positions of nucleus caudalis (Sumino, Nozaki and Katoh, 1981) and in more rostral areas of nucleus oralis and interpolaris (Sessle *et al.*, 1981).

Physiotherapy utilizes massage and functional mobility of the neck, shoulder, limb and jaw muscles in management of CMDs and some physiotherapists now specialize in jaw and cervical muscle problems. In order to provide comprehensive treatment we must acknowledge these interrelationships to correctly diagnose CMDs.

(b) Signs and symptoms

A number of studies of adolescents (Nilner, 1981; Nilner and Lassing, 1981; Wänman and Agerberg, 1986a,b) and adults (Kopp, 1982; Mejersjö, 1984; Carlsson, 1984; Wedel, 1988) have examined the prevalence of signs and symptoms and methods of management of functional disturbances (CMD). In her study of over 300 teenagers, Nilner (1981) found a higher prevalence of symptoms in young adults than amongst children, and Carlsson (1984) has confirmed a higher incidence of CMD in adults.

Epidemiological studies carried out in several countries were reviewed by Carlsson (1984). He confirmed that there was general agreement on the frequency of signs and symptoms amongst patients examined, and that a widespread occurrence of symptoms was identified in non-patient populations.

Longitudinal studies (Wänman, 1987; Wedel, 1988) have reported on the broad variety of signs and symptoms that present in different individuals and the fluctuating nature of their severity.

Table 2.13 is a summary of the clinical features from international studies of CMDs reviewed by Carlsson (1984), who reported the ratio of presenting symptoms to clinical signs as approximately 1:2. That is, many

Table 2.13 Summary of clinical signs and symptoms of CMDs (from Carlsson, 1984)

Clinical signs	(average %)	Presenting symptoms	(average %)
TM joint sounds	26	TM joint sounds	19
tenderness	14	Headache	17
Jaw muscle tenderness	33	Jaw stiffness	11
Jaw movement – pain	4	Jaw movement – pain	6
limited	7	limited	8
		Jaw locking	4

patients examined were unaware of the extent of their clinical signs of CMDs and this relates to illness behaviour or the motivation to seek treatment, the patient's understanding of the problem and their concerns about it.

(c) Clinical signs

Pain originating in the TM joint(s) and due to structural and biomechanical changes within the joint is TM joint pain – dysfunction and presents with:
– pain in the joint(s) and pre-auricular area;
– articular sounds – popping, clicking or grating;
– limited jaw opening and lateral movements;
– radiographic evidence of:
  – alterations in form of the articular fossa, eminence and condyle; and/or
  – alterations in condyle position.

2.5.2 Aetiology

There is increasing clinical, experimental and epidemiological evidence acknowledging the importance of factors other than tooth contact interferences in the aetiology of CMDs (see reviews by Ash, 1986; Zarb and Carlsson, 1988; Clark, Mohl and Riggs, 1988).

It is generally considered that CMDs have a complex aetiology (Franks, 1964; Zarb and Speck, 1977; Kopp, 1982; Hansson, 1988; Wedel, 1988; Mongini, Ventricelli and Conserva, 1988). This writer acknowledges the obvious interrelationship of physical, behavioural and psychological factors in susceptible individuals that contribute to chronic CMDs (see earlier sections of this chapter).

However, the term 'multi-factorial aetiology', which is often used, indicates uncertainty and this writer believes it should not be used without explanation, in describing features of acute CMDs.

A number of general clinical procedures for assessment of CMDs are required during initial assessment and early management. They include jaw muscle and TM joint assessment and tooth alignment and contact features and are described elsewhere (Klineberg, 1991).

Table 2.14 categorizes specific morphofunctional features of the TM joints that must be considered in differential diagnosis of CMDs, and considered in conjunction with possible muscle factors as described in Section 2.4 of this chapter.

Specific features of TM joint dysfunction listed in Table 2.14 are joint sounds, limited mobility and deviation with opening; and an approach to management of these dysfunctions is indicated.

(a) Deviations in form develop as a result of articular loading and remodelling and may result in a click with jaw opening and closing that occurs at the same position in each movement; there is no deviation and no restricted opening.

(b) Eminence click occurs with a deliberate protruded jaw opening in conjunction with a steep posterior slope of the articular tubercle. It is loud and painless and occurs in the middle to late stage of protruded jaw opening. It may be associated with orthodontic treatment, and is often provoked by young patients to 'test' the click for the benefit of their peers. Figure 2.4 shows the profile of a young patient (female, 18 years of age) with an eminence click associated with a protruded jaw opening path – 2.4(2); the click was eliminated with conscious effort to avoid protrusion during opening – 2.4(3).

Table 2.14 Management of TM joint pain (Adapted from Hansson, 1988)

Dysfunction		Clinical signs	Management
Click (soft) associated with deviation in form of condyle	O _‑|‑ ‑ ‑ C / ↓ Max.	Opening and closing click in same position in opening and closing movement	1. Counselling to minimize parafunction 2. Occlusal splint
Click (soft) associated with neuromuscular dysfunction	O _|_ / ↓ Max.	Opening click at a variable position in opening	1. Counselling to minimize parafunction 2. Jaw resistance exercises
Eminence click (hard)	O _|_ / ↓ Max.	Opening click middle to late in opening	1. Jaw resistance exercises 2. Counselling to avoid provoking click
Click (soft) associated with hypermobility	O _|_ / ↓ Max.	Opening click late	1. Occlusal splint 2. Jaw resistance exercises
Click (reciprocal) with anterior disc displacement: Acute → acute pain	O _‑|‑ ‑ ‑C / ↓ Max.	Opening click early Closing click late	1. Manipulation, analgesics 2. Occlusal splint 3. Jaw resistance exercises
Click (reciprocal) with anterior disc displacement: Chronic → mild to no pain	O ‑‑|‑ ‑ ‑ ‑ C / ↓ Max.	Opening click later Closing click earlier	1. Repositioning appliance (6 months) 2. Arthrography 3. Stabilize 3.1 Occlusal adjustment 3.2. Orthodontics/ prosthodontics

Table 2.14 (*Continued*)

Dysfunction		Clinical signs	Management
Anterior disc displacement: Closed – lock Acute Pain severe	O Max.	Opening markedly restricted, deviation to affected side	1. Manipulation, analgesics 2. Repositioning appliance with adjustment over 3 months into occlusal splint for further 3 months 3. Jaw resistance exercises 4. Occlusal adjustment
Anterior disc displacement: Closed – lock Chronic No pain	O Max.	Opening moderately restricted, deviation to affected side	1. Manipulation not possible 2. Unloading appliance, arthrography 3. Physiotherapy 4. Arthroscopy – lysis and lavage 5. Orthodontics/ prosthodontics
Traumatic arthritis – acute hypomobility Acute pain	O Max.	Opening markedly restricted, deviation to affected side	1. Moist heat, rest, analgesics 2. Soft diet 3. Gradual increase in jaw movement 4. May need jaw mobilization exercises
Traumatic arthritis – chronic hypomobility associated with post-traumatic fibrous adhesions No pain	O Max.	Opening restricted (variable), deviation to affected side	1. Mobilization – physiotherapy 2. Arthroscopy – lysis and lavage 3. Occlusal splint 4. Orthodontics, prosthodontics
Degenerative Joint Disease (arthrosis) with periodic acute (arthritis) exacerbations → acute pain	Max.	Opening uneven crepitation with joint movement	1. Unloading appliance (6 months), analgesics 2. Stabilize at increased vertical dimension with prosthodontics 3. Arthrography – may have a perforated disc, may require surgery

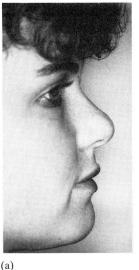
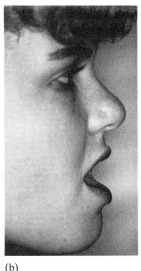
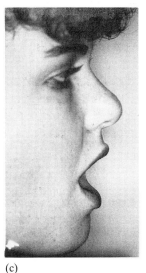

(a) (b) (c)

Figure 2.4 Eminence click.
Eminence click in a young patient (female, 18 years of age) with a history of clicking with pain and parafunctional clenching. The acute pain resolved but the loud click remained. It was provoked as a single click with jaw opening and there was no click on closing. Examination of jaw opening (see (a) and (b)) indicated a marked protruded component of opening which had become a habit, initially to overcome the joint pain.

With training to ensure that jaw opening occurred along a more retrusive path, as in (c), the click was eliminated. Conscious effort was required initially to avoid the protrusive opening path and this was reinforced with isokinetic exercises. An occlusal splint was provided for night use to manage the parafunctional clenching

(c) Hypermobility arises as a result of stretch of discal and articular ligaments and presents as a click occurring late in the opening movement in an older patient, particularly where there is an absence of posterior teeth that has led to progressive changes at the joint.

(d) Acute anterior disc displacement of short duration with acute symptoms of pain. The opening click occurs early and closing click late and there is minimal displacement and distortion of disc and attachment tissues. Pain arises from compression of displaced synovial and attachment tissues.

(e) Chronic anterior disc displacement of long duration where pain symptoms are mild or absent. Opening click occurs later and closing click earlier, suggesting a greater distortion of disc, discal ligaments and attachment tissues of the disc. In this case when the patient protrudes the jaw and opens from a protruded position, the reciprocal click is eliminated.

(f) Anterior disc displacement with acute closed-lock. Jaw opening is markedly restricted, there is deviation to the affected side and acute pain with attempts to open the jaw further. The central bearing surface of the disc has most probably become displaced anteromedially with compression of posterior attachment tissues of the disc.

(g) Anterior disc displacement with chronic closed-lock. In this situation, the opening is moderately restricted with deviation to the affected side. The disc and attachment tissues have become stretched and distorted as a result of long-term displacement of the central bearing surface.

(h) Traumatic arthritis – acute hypomobility and acute pain. In this situation there has been an immediate traumatic incident such as a blow to jaw or face, a fall, motor vehicle accident or the like, with injury to articular soft tissues, particularly the posterior articular tissues. There is a marked restriction in jaw opening with deviation to the affected side and acute pain.

(i) Traumatic arthritis – chronic hypomobility associated with post-traumatic fibrous adhesions; there is no pain. Hypomobility following trauma where there is soft-tissue damage associated with fibrous adhesions that markedly restricts jaw mobility.

(j) Degenerative joint disease, i.e. arthrosis with acute episodes of arthritis. Jaw opening is uneven and there is crepitation with joint movement. The presence of crepitus confirms degenerative joint disease with irreversible changes in articular tissues.

2.5.3 Management – general approach

Acute as well as chronic TM joint dysfunctions are managed conservatively in the first instance. Non-surgical management of CMD involving the TM joints is indicated for the majority (more than 98%) of these problems. Under normal circumstances a surgical approach would only be contemplated following comprehensive conservative therapy. The exception to this general rule is in the case of severe trauma where irreversible damage to articular tissues does not or is unlikely to respond to conservative management.

Table 2.15 lists the treatment possibilities suggested for non-surgical management of CMDs by the American Dental Association President's Conference (Griffiths, 1983). This meeting was the first of its kind to address the problem that the American Dental Association recognized, where a variety of irreversible treatments (such as repositioning appliances, occlusal adjustment, prosthodontic restoration, orthodontic treatment and the like) were being offered to patients in the absence of long-term clinical research designed to assess the efficacy of many of the procedures employed.

The guideline for management of CMDs was explicit in its recommendation:

> 'On the basis of the literature reviews presented . . . it was concluded that at present there is insufficient data to permit comparison of different forms of therapy to establish a priority for their use. However, the basic principle of using conservative reversible forms of therapy, whenever possible, was advocated. Moreover, it was emphasized that a warm, positive, and reassuring attitude on the part of the dentist is crucial in the treatment of these disorders.'

A number of long-term studies have examined the natural history of CMDs and have confirmed the presence of exacerbations and remissions as a feature of these conditions and the value of a conservative approach to management (Franks, 1965a; Rasmussen, 1983; Riise, 1983; Wenneberg, 1983; Hansson, Petersson and Vallon-Christersson, 1984; Dählström, 1984; Mejersjö, 1984; Wedel, 1988).

(a) Palpation
Palpation of lateral and posterolateral areas of the joint both externally and via the external ear canal may elicit tenderness suggesting the presence of articular inflammation with capsulitis and/or synovitis.

Table 2.15 Management of craniomandibular disorders (Adapted from Griffiths 1983, Am. D. A. President's Conference Recommendations*)

1. PHARMACOLOGY – short-term use of appropriate drugs.

2. OCCLUSAL ADJUSTMENT
   – is irreversible treatment;
   – not recommended for routine use, and especially not during acute stages of a TM joint disorder.

3. OCCLUSAL SPLINTS
   – those designed not to alter jaw position have reversible effects;
   – these appliances are recommended;
   – scientific evidence exists for their efficacy.

4. REPOSITIONING APPLIANCES
   – intentional permanent placement of jaw in new position is irreversible treatment;*
   – jaw repositioning appliances may be considered reversible unless followed by:
     occlusal adjustment, prosthetic restoration,
     orthodontic treatment, surgical treatment.
   – scientific evidence supporting this treatment* is not available.

5. PHYSICAL THERAPY
   – is reversible treatment.

6. SURGERY
   – arthroscopy may be regarded as benign, minimally invasive surgery and includes lysis and lavage (this author has added this procedure as it is now routinely used);
   – indicated for developmental and acquired abnormalities, ankylosis, neoplasia;
   – functional disorders do not warrant surgery;
   – there is no evidence for surgery in initial treatment of disc displacement problems;
   – only after failure of conservative treatment should surgery be considered, and then only when based on definite criteria for surgery;
   – there is little support for menisectomy.

7. OSTEOPATHIC, CHIROPRACTIC TREATMENT
   – supporting evidence for the efficacy of the treatments does not exist.

* Griffiths, R. H. (1983) Report of the President's Conference on the examination, diagnosis and management of temporomandibular disorders. *Journal of the American Dental Association*, **106**, 75–77.

(b) Medication
Anti-inflammatory agents are of value in providing specific short-term treatment for acute inflammation of articular tissues. Symptomatic relief may be provided by analgesic (see Table 2.11), however aspirin is special in that as well as its analgesic effects, it is also anti-inflammatory for joint tissues. If this is not appropriate, other non-steroid anti-inflammatory agents are available (Table 2.16).

(c) Articular nerve block
Local anaesthetic block of the articular branches of the auriculotemporal nerve is of diagnostic value (Klineberg and Lillie, 1980; Kreisberg, 1986).

Table 2.16 Non-steroid anti-inflammatory agents

Active component	Proprietary name	Manufacturer
Aspirin	Bi-Prin (650 mg) Sig. 2 tabs b.d.	Boots
	Bufferin (325 mg with magnesium carbonate 97.2 mg, aluminium glycinate 48.6 mg) Sig. 1–3 tabs q.i.d.	Astra
	Ecotrin (650 mg)	Smith, Kline & French
	SRA (650 mg) Sig. 3 tabs b.d.	Boots
	Winsprin (325 mg)	Winthrop
Diclofenac sodium	Voltaren Sig. 25 mg t.i.d. up to 150 mg daily in divided doses	Ciba-Geigy
Ibuprofen	Brufen (400 mg) Sig. 1200 mg in 3 divided doses	Boots
	Inflam (200, 400 mg) Sig. 400 mg t.i.d.	Protea
Indomethacin	Indocid (25 mg) Sig. 50–200 mg daily after meals	Merck Sharp & Dohme
	Rheumacin (25 mg) Sig. 25–50 mg t.i.d. with food	Protea
Naproxen	Naprosyn (250 mg) Sig. 250 mg b.d. up to max. of 750 mg/day	Syntex

If pain originates primarily from within the joint, regional nerve block will induce temporary relief of symptoms.

This may occur either as a result of regional anaesthesia of articular tissues *per se*, or from the reflex effects on jaw muscles (Greenfield and Wyke, 1966) following anaesthetic block of mechanoreceptors in the articular capsule, which inhibits their afferent activity. If the problem is primarily of muscular origin, it will remain unaltered after regional nerve block of articular tissues.

(d) Physiotherapy (see Table 2.12)
A number of procedures are appropriate for management of acute TM joint dysfunction (Hargreaves and Wardle, 1983) in a similar manner to that used for management of acute muscle problems (see Section 2.4.4). Heat is indicated for acute traumatic arthritis and this may be supported with ultrasound or short-wave diathermy to increase vascularity and assist resolution of inflammation. Mobilization (stretch–relax) exercises are recommended for hypomobility associated with a previous traumatic episode leading to the formation of fibrous adhesions. Resistance or isokinetic exercises are used to strengthen jaw muscles by retraining extensor and flexor muscles. Figure 2.5 and the instruction for patients

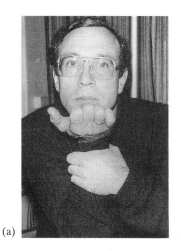
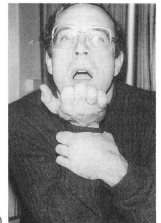

(a)

(b)

Figure 2.5 (a) and (b) Frontal view of patient seated in the correct manner for carrying out the series of open-close isokinetic exercises. The patient's right hand supports the chin whilst the left hand helps to stabilize the right arm, and the elbow rests on a firm surface. Jaw opening is carried out against the resistance of the hand over a hinge movement in order to avoid joint translation. In this way, open-close movements, if restricted to less than 20 mm inter-incisor separation, will avoid provoking pain or clicking. This exercise sequence is repeated twenty times morning and night.

(c) and (d) Lateral view of the above.

(e) and (f) Lateral exercises carried out against the support of the hand. The extent of lateral movements is 5 mm to avoid provoking a click. Lateral isokinetic exercises are performed ten times morning and night

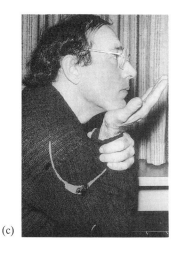
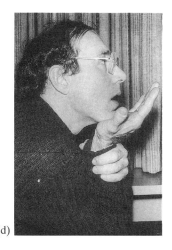

(c)

(d)

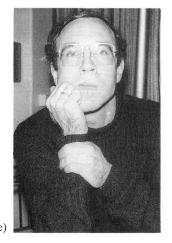
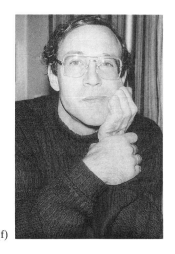

(e)

(f)

(shown in Appendix III) clearly indicate the manner in which these exercises are carried out.

Isokinetic exercises (Basmajian, 1979) are designed to allow controlled joint movement under continuous load (resistance) with simultaneous activity of extensor and flexor muscles operating about the joint. Such exercises are appropriate for limb and postural joints as well as jaw joints, and are designed to retrain and strengthen the muscle system moving the joint. Movement is restricted to avoid provoking discomfort, pain or joint sounds.

Hislop and Perrine (1967) compared the different exercise therapies as used in physical medicine:

(i) Isotonic exercise is where the joint is moved through a range (usually with weights) of motion with constant resistance, but where muscle resistance varies and is greatest at the extremes of movement. Thus tension demand on a muscle is at a maximum only over a small part of the movement range. With the jaw muscle system, isotonic exercise occurs with open-close and lateral jaw movement.

(ii) Isometric exercise is where resistance is sufficient to prevent joint movement, allowing the muscles to develop maximum load in one joint position.

With the jaw muscle system, isometric exercise occurs with the jaw in IP with muscle clenching, as occurs in 'centric' bruxism, or in an eccentric jaw position (often anterolateral) where tooth contact on bruxofacets provide a firm area of contact (eccentric bruxism).

(iii) Isokinetic exercise is joint movement by muscle contraction with an external means of controlling the speed of movement. In physical medicine a suitable mechanical device is used to load the system and control speed of joint movement. This promotes the full muscle force potential of the particular joint system throughout a range of motion.

With the jaw muscle system, chin resistance allows controlled jaw open-close and lateral movements over a restricted range of motion allowing full activity of all muscles operating about the joint.

The exercise sequence for the jaw joint (Figure 2.6) requires movement against a resistance (Berman and Klineberg, 1982; Au and Klineberg, 1989) as follows:

Jaw open-close	(twenty times)
Jaw to right	(ten times)
Jaw to left	(ten times)

This sequence is carried out morning and night.

Resistance may be provided by placing the palm of the hand against the chin (Figure 2.6) with the arm stabilized and the elbow resting against a firm surface, or by holding the clenched hand against the chin with the arm firmly pressed against the chest.

These exercises are indicated in the management of painless clicking or once a painful episode has resolved, and where the click is not caused by a displaced interarticular disc. Berman and Klineberg (1982) and Au and

Klineberg (1989) found that in their controlled studies, two-thirds of the painless clicks resolved within a month with isokinetic exercises and at follow-up one year after completing the exercise sequence, 19 of the 20 subjects remained free of their click.

The exercise sequence is appropriate for all age groups, and speed of recovery depends on the duration of the dysfunction and thus the integrity of the interarticular disc. When the central bearing surface of the disc has been damaged and the posterior elastic fibres injured by a permanent relocation of the disc anterior to the condyle, then exericse therapy is unlikely to be effective. However, it is of particular value in children and young adults, where the condyle-disc derangement is of short duration.

(e) Imaging

A number of approaches to TM joint imaging are now available depending on whether the need is to visualize bone (condyle, eminence) or soft tissue (interarticular disc). The following briefly describes these possibilities:

(i) Panoramic radiographs are valuable for general screening. The orthopantomographic (OPT) technique can be modified to clearly visualize coronoid process, articular tubercle and condyle. With the patient positioned forward of the standard position, and by lowering the chin slightly and opening the patient's mouth, an improved view of the joints is obtained. OPT views of the TM joints show general morphological features bilaterally, such a relative size and shape of the condyle, the presence of surface contour changes reflecting deviations in form and possibly degenerative changes.

Such views do not provide information about joint position or details of degenerative changes. However, clinical studies by Hansson (1988), Bezuur, Habets and Hansson (1989), Bezuur, Hansson and Wilkinson (1989) indicate that the OPT is valuable in establishing a preliminary diagnosis of a CMD. The presence of a significant vertical condylar height asymmetry suggests a myogenous or arthrogenous pain problem and requires comprehensive clinical assessment.

(ii) Lateral transcranial radiographs provide more accurate visualization of the profile of the TM joint, but should be standardized and corrected. Standardized transcranial lateral views may be useful in making an assessment of condyle position. Transcranial lateral views are a two-dimensional representation of a three-dimensional object of highly variable morphology. Thus, if any value is to be placed on transcranial TM joint radiographs, either as to the presence of pathology, or to condyle position, a standardized radiographic technique is essential.

Standardized procedures requires a TM joint cephalostat* to orientate precisely the incident X-ray beam with respect to the condyle to minimize overlap of structures. It also allows radiographs that have been taken on

---

*Some varieties of cephalostats available:
  Updegrave, W. J. – Fort Lauderdale, FL 33307, USA;
  Buhner, W. A. – Daytona Beach, FL 32018, USA;
  Accurad 100 – Denar Corp., Anaheim, CA 92805, USA;
  Graf – TMX: Andre Vaudaux AG, Basel, Switzerland.

different occasions to be compared as a means of monitoring the progress of treatment.

Corrected transcranial radiographs require a preliminary submentovertex projection to indicate the orientation of the long axis of the condyle. The angle of the long axis of the condyle with the horizontal plane is measured and the incident X-ray beam may then be adjusted to be aligned along the long axis of the condyle. Such transcranial views are suitable for detecting bony arthroses, changes in articular form and providing an indication of the spatial position of the lateral one-third of the condyle. The latter information may be of value when correlated with clinical assessment (Klineberg, 1991).

(iii) Transpharyngeal projection. This technique was refined by Toller (Toller, 1969, Ogus and Toller, 1981) for use with a standard dental X-ray unit in the dental surgery without the need for a cephalostat. The patient is seated upright with the mouth open 2 cm and anterior teeth gently biting on an incisal support.

The jaw opening allows the X-ray beam to be directed through the sigmoid notch, across the pharynx towards the medial pole of the contralateral condyle. TM joint radiographs without the superimposition of bony structures may be obtained in this way.

A concern with this technique is the relatively long exposure required.

(iv) Tomography provides unique sectional views of joint structures allowing pathological changes and more detailed morphological changes to be assessed. The visualization of sections of articular components avoids superimposition of structures and reveals greater detail of hard tissue changes. The width of the sectional view varies with the specifications of the X-ray tube and the anatomy of the object, and is of the order of 3 mm for the TM joint. The principle of obtaining a sectional view depends on the simultaneous movement of the X-ray tube and X-ray film in opposite directions, with the axis of rotation at the object to be visualized. In this way the area required is sharply defined, whilst areas on either side are blurred.

Different forms of tomography are available depending on the pattern of movement of tube and film – the commonest ones are linear (straight), circular (curved-circular path), ellipsoid (curved elliptical path) and hypocycloidal (complex clover-leaf path). Rosenberg and Silha (1982) have comprehensively reviewed TM joint radiography with special emphasis on tomography, and clearly describe and illustrate these different approaches.

Linear tomography should be corrected to provide the axial orientation of the long axis of the condyle. As before, a submentovertex projection is necessary to provide the details of condylar axial inclination. This then allows the tomographic sections to be made at right angles to the long axis of the condyle. Each joint is considered separately, as the orientation of the condyle long axis may be significantly different on each side. Lateral and frontal tomographic views may be made to show the profile and frontal view of the joint.

Petersson (1987) reported that the need for corrected linear tomography is important to minimize distortion. With hypocycloidal tomography, however, divergencies of beam angle to condyle long axis of up to 15× do not affect the image. The more complex movement pattern reduces superimposition errors and distortions. The need for tomographic views is determined by the complexity of the case and the appropriateness of the information obtained from simpler radiographic procedures. Rohlin, Åkerman and Kopp (1986) confirmed the accuracy of corrected tomography in identifying macroscopic changes in articular tissues and that changes in the condyle were more readily detected than changes in the temporal component.

(v) Arthrography requires the introduction of a radio-opaque water soluble contrast medium (as with double contrast tomography) into the lower joint space alone or into the lower followed by the upper compartment. Immediately following the introduction of contrast, transcranial or tomographic views are made with the jaw closed and open. The injection of contrast medium into the lower joint compartment will clearly define the inferior surface of the interarticular disc and indicate the location of its central bearing surface. Disc perforation is clearly revealed by the passage of contrast into the upper joint compartment. Arthrography is being used extensively now in differential diagnosis of internal derangements to determine whether the interarticular disc is displaced, the degree of displacement, the feasibility of reducing the displacement (Farrar and McCarty, 1979; Tallens *et al.*, 1986; Roberts *et al.*, 1987a) and the need for surgery (Wilkes, 1978a,b; McCarty and Farrar, 1979; Bronstein, Tomasetti and Ryan, 1981). The use of arthrography in differential diagnosis, particularly for chronic disorders unresponsive to conservative treatment, is an asset as it provides an additional dimension to clinical assessment. Correlation of arthrographic findings and clinical assessment has confirmed the unreliability of clinical assessment alone in diagnosis and monitoring of treatment. The need and value of arthrography, particularly in management of internal derangements to ensure an optimum condyle-disc relationship, has been emphasized (Manzione *et al.*, 1984; Laney *et al.*, 1987; Roberts *et al.*, 1987a,b).

(vi) Other imaging procedures are available such as bone scintigraphy (Epstein and Ruprecht, 1982), computed tomography, CT (Christiansen *et al.*, 1987) and magnetic resonance imaging, MRI (Sanchez-Woodworth *et al.*, 1988). The more sophisticated imaging procedures have exciting possibilities in providing details of internal structures that were not previously possible. The need for specialist radiographic support is obvious and emphasizes the requirement for a multidisciplinary approach in order to provide optimum patient care.

(f) Intra-articular injections
Injection of anti-inflammatory medication into the joint space may be considered in acute inflammatory conditions:

1. Acute rheumatic arthritis
2. Acute exacerbation of degenerative joint disease
3. Acute intra-articular inflammation

A 50% mixture of hydrocortisone (50–100 mg), a-methazone or prednisolone (25–50 mg) together with 50% lignocaine (plain), has been shown to be particularly beneficial (Wenneberg and Kopp, 1978).

However, such procedures are likely to result in disc degeneration. This has become apparent following the routine use of arthroscopy and intra-articular injection of anti-inflammatory medication are no longer recommended.

2.5.4 Management – specific approach

Table 2.14 summarizes the specific treatment procedures required for the management of diagnosed morphofunctional disorders.

(a) Click associated with deviation in form
Management requires occlusal splint therapy to provide temporary joint unloading to overcome the dysfunction, followed by restorative procedures to maintain the increased vertical dimension of occlusion. Restorations provide permanent unloading of articular tissues to arrest further deterioration and to encourage reparative remodelling.

(b) Eminence click
Management requires resistance or isokinetic exercises to retrain the muscles to avoid the protrusive type of jaw opening. Counselling is needed to explain the mechanism of the click and the way in which it is being provoked; and if it is an attention-seeking mechanism the need to avoid the habit in order to prevent further damage to the tissues of a young joint must be emphasized.

(c) Click associated with hypermobility
Management requires an occlusal splint to reduce the tendency for clicking, a conscious effort to resist excessive mobility in jaw movement and resistance exercises of the jaw to strengthen jaw muscles to better resist hypermobility and encourage remodelling of ligaments.

(d) Click with anterior disc displacement, acute-severe
Management involves analgesics and jaw manipulation (jaw is brought downwards and forwards to distract the joint and bring it forward) to correctly realign disc and condyle (i.e. disc 'recapture'). An occlusal splint is fitted to eliminate guiding tooth inclines that may cause the condyle to be displaced distally in the fossa. Jaw resistance exercises are required to strengthen the jaw muscles.

(e) Click with anterior disc displacement, chronic
Management requires a repositioning appliance constructed to a slightly protruded jaw position, which must be worn continuously day and night for six months. The resolution of symptoms is immediate, and remodelling and repair of articular tissues should occur, arthrography is used to confirm the realignment that might be achieved clinically. The jaw is stabilized to maintain the anterior position after approximately six months by occlusal adjustment, orthodontic extrusion of posterior teeth or prosthodontic treatment.

(f) Anterior disc displacement with acute closed-lock

Manipulation is required as soon as possible to realign disc and condyle and a repositioning appliance (see Chapter 4, Section 4.7) is needed initially to provide support for the traumatized articular tissues and allow posterior joint space for the acute inflammation to resolve. The appliance is adjusted over a period of three months to progressively return the condyle and disc to their original position (or close to this position) and in the process convert the repositioning appliance into a stabilizing occlusal splint. Jaw resistance exercises are desirable to strengthen jaw muscles and an occlusal adjustment may be required. The adjustment would eliminate tooth and cuspal guidance that are seen to encourage a distal jaw displacement at tooth contact (i.e. eliminate plunger cusps, distally directed non-working interferences, distal guidance in lateral excursions, posterior guidance in protrusive excursions and the like).

(g) Anterior disc displacement with chronic closed-lock

Management requires an unloading appliance (see Chapter 4, Section 4.7) since jaw manipulation does not eliminate the disc displacement. After the unloading appliance is fitted, arthrography is used to confirm that the disc is correctly aligned. The appliance is designed to encourage disc and condyle realignment and this may require jaw exercises and physiotherapy. If unsuccessful, manipulation under general anaesthesia will confirm whether realignment is possible or arthroscopy with lysis and lavage is indicated. The continued use of the unloading appliance is necessary. The jaw position would then be stabilized by orthodontic realignment of molar teeth or with prosthodontic treatment where posterior tooth build-up with onlays, crowns or removable appliances would be required.

(h) Traumatic arthritis – acute hypomobility and pain

Management requires a variety of procedures to reduce the inflammation, including moist heat and rest, a soft diet, and a gradual increase in jaw movement as inflammation begins to resolve. There may be a need for jaw mobilization exercises to avoid the development of fibrosis. Mobilization exercises require articular tissues to be stretched with wide opening, lateral and protrusive movements. These exercises are quite different from resistance exercises such as isokinetic exercises, which are designed to strengthen the extensor and flexor muscles of the joint.

(i) Traumatic arthritis – chronic hypomobility without pain

Management requires physiotherapy to increase mobilization and break up adhesions. There may be a need for manipulation under general anaesthetic if physiotherapy is not successful, or arthroscopy with lysis and lavage to remove adhesions. An occlusal splint is desirable following manipulation to stabilize the jaw.

(j) Degenerative joint disease

Management requires an unloading appliance to be used full-time for six months, followed by permanently stabilizing the jaw support at an increased vertical dimension. This condition is likely to involve the older patient where stabilization with prosthodontic treatment is indicated. Arthrography is needed to confirm whether there is a perforated interarticular disc, and whether its surgical removal is required.

(k) Rheumatoid disease

Management of the acute episodes of rheumatoid disease involving the jaw joint requires an unloading appliance to be used full-time. Following the acute phase, the appliance may be removed and optimum function may be possible, depending on the degree of erosion that has occurred at the temporomandibular condyle. There may be a need for more permanent unloading to be provided by fixed splints, crowns or bridges in order to allow full function to return where destruction of the condyle has been excessive. Medical management will also be necessary and treatment should be carried out in conjunction with the patient's medical specialist.

References

Abrahams, V. C. (1977) The physiology of neck muscles; their role in head movement and maintenance of posture. *Canadian Journal of Physiology,* **53**, 332–338

Abrahams, V. C. and Richmond, F. J. R. (1977) Motor role of the spinal projections of the trigeminal system. In *Pain in the Trigeminal Region* (eds D. J. Anderson and B. Matthews), Elsevier/North Holland Biomedical, Amsterdam, pp. 405–411

Anderson, D. J., Hannam, A. C. and Matthews, B. (1970) Sensory mechanisms in mammalian teeth and their supporting structures. *Physiological Reviews,* **50**, 171–195

Ash, M. M. (1986) Current concepts in the aetiology, diagnosis and treatment of TMJ and muscle dysfunction. *Journal of Oral Rehabilitation,* **13**, 1–20

Au, A. and Klineberg, I. (1989) Isokinetic exercise management of temporomandibular clicking. *Journal of Dental Research,* **68** (Abstr. 22): 541

Award, E. A. (1973) Interstitial myofibrositis hypotheses of the mechanism. *Archives of Physical Medicine and Rehabilitation,* **54**, 449–453

Ayer, W. A. (1979) Thumb-fingersucking and bruxing habits in children. In *Oral Motor Behaviour: Impact on Oral Conditions and Dental Treatment* (eds P. Bryant, E. Gale and J. Rugh), NIH Publication 79-1845, pp. 7–23

Bailey, J. O. and Rugh, J. D. (1979) Behavioural management of functional oral disorders. In *Oral Motor Behaviour: Impact on Oral Conditions and Dental Treatment* (eds P. Bryant, E. Gale and J. Rugh), NIH Publication 79-1845, pp. 160–178

Bakke, M., Møller, E. and Thorsen, N. M. (1982) Occlusal control of temporalis and masseter activity during mastication. *Journal of Dental Research,* **61** (Abstr. 704): 257

Basmajian, J. V. (1972) Electromyography comes of age. *Science,* **176**, 603–609

Basmajian, J. V. (1979) *Muscles Alive*, 4th edn, Williams & Wilkins, Baltimore, pp. 83–91, 164–169

Bell, W. E. (1973) *Orofacial Pains – Differential Diagnosis*, Denedco of Dallas, Dallas, pp. 244, 294

Berman, A. and Klineberg, I. (1982) Isokinetic exercise therapy in management of temporomandibular joint dysfunction with clicking. *Journal of Dental Research,* **61**, (Abstr. 52): 529

Berry, D. C. (1969) Mandibular dysfunction and chronic minor stress. *British Dental Journal,* **127**, 170–175

Berry, D. C. and Harris, M. (1985) Medical or physical management of facial muscle and joint pain? *British Dental Journal,* **158**, 227–229

Bezuur, J. N., Habets, L. L. M. H. and Hansson, T. L. (1989) The recognition of craniomandibular disorders – condylar symmetry in relation to myogenous and arthrogenous origin of pain. *Journal of Oral Rehabilitation,* **16**, 257–260

Bezuur, J. N., Hansson, T. L. and Wilkinson, T. M. (1989) The recognition of craniomandibular disorders – an evaluation of the most reliable signs and symptoms when screening for CMD. *Journal of Oral Rehabilitation,* **16**, 367–372

Bogduk, N. (1982) The clinical anatomy of the cervical dorsal rami. *Spine,* **7**, 319–330

Bonde-Petersen, F. and Christensen, L. V. (1973) Blood flow in human temporal muscle during tooth grinding and clenching as measured by [133]Xenon clearance. *Scandinavian Journal of Dental Research,* **81**, 272–275

Brännström, M. (1963) A hydrodynamic mechanism in the transmission of pain-producing stimuli through the dentine. In *Sensory Mechanisms in Dentine* (ed. D. J. Anderson), Pergamon Press, Oxford, pp. 73–79

Brännström, M. (1986) The hydrodynamic theory of dentinal pain: sensation in preparations, caries and the dentinal crack syndrome. *Journal of Endodontics,* **12**, 453–457

Brännström, M. and Åström, A. (1972) The hydrodynamics of dentine; its possible relationship to dentinal pain. *International Dental Journal,* **22**, 219–227

Bray, G. M. and Aguayo, A. J. (1974) Regeneration of peripheral unmyelinated nerves. Fate of the axonal sprouts which develop after injury. *Journal of Anatomy,* **117**, 517–529

Bronstein, S. L., Tomasetti, B. J. and Ryan, D. E. (1981) Internal derangements of the temporomandibular joint: correlation of arthrography with surgical findings. *Journal of Oral Surgery,* **39**, 572–584

Byers, M. R. and Dong, W. K. (1981) Autoradiographic demonstration of sensory nerve endings in monkey teeth. *Pain,* Suppl. 1, S201

Byers, M. R. and Matthews, B. (1981) Autoradiographic demonstration of ipsilateral and contralateral sensory nerve endings in cat dentine, pulp and periodontium. *Anatomical Record,* **201**, 249–260

Carlsson, G. E. (1984) Epidemiological studies of signs and symptoms of temporomandibular joint-pain-dysfunction. A literature review. *Australian Prosthodontic Society Bulletin,* **14**, 7–12

Christiansen, E. L., Thompson, J. R., Zimmerman, G. *et al.* (1987) Computed tomography of condylar and articular disk positions within the temporomandibular joint. *Oral Surgery,* **64**, 757–767

Christensen, L. V. (1970) Facial pain from experimental tooth clenching. *Tandlaeggebladet,* **74**, 175–178

Christensen, L. V. (1971) Facial pain and internal pressure of masseter muscle in experimental bruxism in man. *Archives of Oral Biology,* **16**, 1021–1031

Christensen, L. V. (1979) Influence of muscle pain tolerance on muscle pain threshold in experimental tooth clenching in man. *Journal of Oral Rehabilitation,* **6**, 211–217

Clark, G. T., Mohl, N. D. and Riggs, R. R. (1988) Occlusal adjustment therapy. In *A Textbook of Occlusion* (eds N. D. Mohl, G. A. Zarb, G. E. Carlsson and J. D. Rugh), Quintessence, Chicago, pp. 285–303

Clarke, N. G. and Kardachi, B. J. (1977) The treatment of myofascial pain-dysfunction syndrome using the biofeedback principle. *Journal of Periodontology,* **48**, 643–645

Costen, J. B. (1934) A syndrome of ear and sinus symptoms dependent upon disturbed function of the temporomandibular joint. *Annals of Otology,* **43**, 1–15

Dählström, L. (1984) Conservative treatment of mandibular dysfunction. *Swedish Dental Journal,* Suppl. 24

De Boever, J. A. (1979) Functional disturbances of the temporomandibular joint. In *Temporomandibular Joint Function and Dysfunction* (eds G. A. Zarb and G. E. Carlsson), C. V. Mosby, St Louis, pp. 193–214

Dworkin, S. F. and Burgess, J. A. (1987) Orofacial pain of psychogenic origin: current concepts and classification. *Journal of the American Dental Association,* **115**, 565–571

Elias, S. A., Taylor, A. and Somjen, G. (1987) Direct and relayed projection of periodontal receptor afferents to the cerebellum in the ferrett. *Proceedings of the Royal Society, London,* **B231**, 199–216

Ellis, S., Howell, P. G. T., Johnson, C. J. and Klineberg, I. (1990) The reproducibility of jaw movement in normal subjects. *Journal of Dental Research,* **69** (Abstr. 111): 946

Epstein, J. B. and Ruprecht, A. (1982) Bone scintigraphy: An aid in diagnosis and management of facial pain associated with osteoarthrosis. *Oral Surgery,* **53**, 37–42

Eriksson, P. O. and Thornell, L. E. (1983) Histochemical and morphological muscle-fibre characteristics of the human masseter, the medial pterygoid and the temporal muscles. *Archives of Oral Biology,* **28**, 781–795

Farrar, W. B. and McCarty, W. L. (1979) Inferior joint space arthrography and characteristics of condylar paths in internal derangements of the TMJ. *Journal of Prosthetic Dentistry,* **41**, 548–555

Fearnhead, R. W. (1963) The histological demonstration of nerve fibres in human dentine. In *Sensory Mechanisms in Dentine* (ed. D. J. Anderson), Pergamon Press, Oxford, pp. 15–26

Feine, J. S., Hutchins, M. O. and Lund, J. P. (1988) An evaluation of the criteria used to diagnose mandibular dysfunction with the mandibular kinesiograph. *Journal of Prosthetic Dentistry,* **60**, 374–380

Feinmann, C. (1985) Pain relief by antidepressants: possible modes of action. *Pain,* **23**, 1–8

Feinmann, C. and Harris, M. (1984a) Psychogenic facial pain Part 1: the clinical presentation. *British Dental Journal,* **156**, 165–168

Feinmann, C. and Harris, M. (1984b) Psychogenic facial pain Part 2: management and prognosis. *British Dental Journal,* **156**, 205–208

Fosberg, C.-M., Hellsing, E., Linder-Aronson, S. and Sheikholeslam, A. (1985) EMG activity in neck and masticatory muscles in relation to extension and flexion of the head. *European Journal of Orthodontics,* **7**, 177–184

Frank, R. M. (1968) Ultra structural relationship between the odontoblast, its process and the nerve fibre. In *Dentine and Pulp: Their Structure and Reactions* (ed. N. B. B. Symonds), Livingstone, Edinburgh, pp. 115–146

Franks, A. S. T. (1964) The social character of temporomandibular joint dysfunction. *Dental Practitioner and Dental Record,* **15**, 94–100

Franks, A. S. T. (1965a) Conservative treatment of temporomandibular joint dysfunction: a comparative study. *Dental Practitioner and Dental Record,* **15**, 205–210

Franks, A. S. T. (1965b) Masticatory muscle hyperactivity and temporomandibular joint dysfunction. *Journal of Prosthetic Dentistry,* **15**, 1112–1131

Garberoglio, R. and Brännström, M. (1976) Scanning electron microscopical investigation of human dentinal tubules. *Archives of Oral Biology,* **21**, 355–362

Goldstein, I. B. (1964) Role of muscle tension in personality theory. *Psychological Bulletin,* **61**, 413–425

Goodman, P., Greene, C. S. and Laskin, D. M. (1976) Response of patients with myofascial pain-dysfunction syndrome to mock equilibration. *Journal of the American Dental Association,* **92**, 755–758

Greene, C. S. (1973) A survey of current professional concepts and opinions about the myofascial pain-dysfunction (MPD) syndrome. *Journal of the American Dental Association,* **86**, 128–136

Greene, C. S. and Laskin, D. M. (1972) Splint therapy for the myofascial pain-dysfunction (MPD) syndrome: a comparative study. *Journal of the American Dental Association,* **84**, 624–628

Greene, C. S. and Laskin, D. M. (1974) Long-term evaluation of conservative treatment for myofascial pain-dysfunction syndrome. *Journal of the American Dental Association,* **89**, 1365–1368

Greene, C. S., Olson, R. E. and Laskin, D. M. (1982) Psychological factors in the etiology, progression, and treatment of MPD syndrome. *Journal of the American Dental Association,* **105**, 443–448

Greenfield, B. E. and Wyke, B. (1966) Reflex innervation of the temporomandibular joint. *Nature,* **211**, 940–941

Gregg, J. M. (1971) Post-traumatic pain: experimental trigeminal neuropathy. *Journal of Oral Surgery,* **29**, 260–267

Gregg, J. M. (1978) Post-traumatic trigeminal neuralgia: response to physiologic, surgical and pharmacologic therapies. *International Dental Journal,* **28**, 43–51

Griffiths, R. H. (1983) Report of the President's Conference on the examination, diagnosis and management of temporomandibular disorders. *Journal of the American Dental Association,* **106**, 75–77

Gunji, T. (1982) Morphological research on the sensitivity of dentin. *Archivum Histologicum Japonicum,* **45**, 45–67

Hansson, L.-G., Petersson, A. and Vallon-Christersson, D. (1984) Clinical and radiologic six-year follow-up study of patients with crepitation of the temporomandibular joint. *Swedish Dental Journal*, **8**, 277–287

Hansson, T. L. (1988) Craniomandibular disorders and sequencing their treatment. *Australian Prosthodontic Journal*, **2**, 9–15

Hargreaves, A. S. and Wardle, J. J. M. (1983) The use of physiotherapy in the treatment of temporomandibular disorders. *British Dental Journal*, **155**, 121–123

Harris, M. (1974) Psychogenic aspects of facial pain. *British Dental Journal*, **136**, 199–202

Harris, R. and Griffin, C. J. (1968) Fine structure of nerve endings in the human dental pulp. *Archives of Oral Biology*, **13**, 773–778

Helkimo, M. (1976) Epidemiological surveys of dysfunction of the masticatory system. *Oral Sciences Reviews*, **7**, 54–69

Hellsing, E. (1987) Craniofacial morphology related to body and head posture. *Doctorate Thesis*, School of Dentistry, Karolinska Institute, Stockholm

Hellsing, E., Reigo, T., McWilliam, J. and Spangfort, E. (1987) Cervical and lumbar lordosis and thoracic kyphosis in 8, 11 and 15 year old children. *European Journal of Orthodontics*, **9**, 1–10

Hellsing, G. and Lindström, L. (1983) Rotation of synergistic activity during isometric jaw muscle contraction in man. *Acta Physiologica Scandinavica*, **118**, 203–207

Hislop, H. J. and Perrine, J. J. (1967) The isokinetic concept of exercise. *Physical Therapy*, **47**, 114–117

Howe, J. F. (1983) Phantom limb pain – a re-afferentation syndrome. *Pain*, **15**, 101–107

Johnsen, D. C., Harshbarger, J. and Rymer, H. D. (1983) Quantitative assessment of neural development in human premolars. *Anatomical Record*, **205**, 421–429

Kardachi, B. J. and Clarke, N. G. (1977) The use of biofeedback to control bruxism. *Journal of Periodontology*, **48**, 639–642

Kent, G. (1985) Memory of dental pain. *Pain*, **21**, 187–194

Klineberg, I. (1991) *Occlusion: Principles and Assessment*, Butterworth-Heinemann, Oxford

Klineberg, I. and Lillie, J. (1980) Regional nerve block of the temporomandibular joint capsule: A technique for clinical research and differential diagnosis. *Journal of Dental Research*, **59**, 1930–1935

Kopp, S. (1982) Pain and functional disturbances of the masticatory system – a review of etiology and principles of treatment. *Swedish Dental Journal*, **6**, 49–60

Kraus, H. (1969) Physical methods. In *Facial Pain and Mandibular Dysfunction* (eds L. Schwartz and C. M. Chayes), W. B. Saunders, Philadelphia, pp. 281–299

Kreisberg, M. K. (1986) Headache as a symptom of craniomandibular disorders II: management. *Journal of Craniomandibular Practice*, **4**, 220–228

Krogh-Poulsen, W. and Olsson, A. (1969) Management of the occlusion of the teeth. In *Facial Pain and Mandibular Dysfunction* (eds L. Schwartz and C. M. Chayes), W. B. Saunders, Philadelphia, pp. 236–280

Laney, T. J., Kaplan, P. A., Tu, H. K. and Lydiatt, D. D. (1987) Normal and abnormal temporomandibular joints: quantitative evaluation of inferior joint space arthrography. *International Journal of Oral and Maxillofacial Surgery*, **16**, 305–311

Laskin, D. M. (1969) Etiology of the pain-dysfunction syndrome. *Journal of the American Dental Association*, **79**, 147–153

Lehmann, J. F., Delateur, B. J., Warren, C. G. and Stonebridge, J. B. (1968) Heating of joint structures by ultrasound. *Archives of Physical Medicine*, **49**, 28–30

Lilja, J. (1979) Innervation of the different parts of the predentin and dentin in young human premolars. *Acta Odontologica Scandinavica*, **37**, 339–346

Lund, J. P. and Widmer, C. G. (1989) An evaluation of the use of surface electromyography in the diagnosis, documentation, and treatment of dental patients. *Journal of Craniomandibular Disease Facial and Oral Pain*, **3**, 125–137

Lupton, D. E. (1969) Psychological aspects of temporomandibular joint dysfunction. *Journal of the American Dental Association*, **79**, 131–136

Mahan, P. E. (1975) Temporomandibular joint dysfunction: physiological and clinical aspects. In *Occlusion Research in Form and Function* (ed. N. H. Rowe), Symposium: University of Michigan

Malow, R. M., Grimm, L. and Olson, R. E. (1980) Differences in pain perception between myofascial pain dysfunction patients and normal subjects: a signal detection analysis. *Journal of Psychosomatic Research*, **24**, 303–309

Manzione, J. V., Tallens, R., Katzberg, R. W. *et al.* (1984) Arthrographically guided splint therapy for recapturing the temporomandibular joint meniscus. *Oral Surgery,* **57**, 235–240

Marbach, J. J. (1976) Phantom bite. *American Journal of Orthodontics,* **70**, 190–199

Marbach, J. J. (1977) Arthritis of the temporomandibular joint and facial pain. *Bulletin of Rheumatic Diseases,* **27**, 918–921

Marbach, J. J. (1978a) Phantom bite syndrome. *American Journal of Psychiatry,* **135**, 476–479

Marbach, J. J. (1978b) Phantom tooth pain. *Journal of Endodontics,* **4**, 362–372

Marbach, J. J. and Lipton, J. A. (1978) Aspects of illness behaviour in patients with facial pain. *Journal of the American Dental Association,* **96**, 630–637

Marbach, J. J., Varoscak, J. R. and Blank, R. T. (1983) 'Phantom bite': classification and treatment. *Journal of Prosthetic Dentistry,* **49**, 556–559

McCarty, W. L. and Farrar, W. B. (1979) Surgery for internal derangements of the temporomandibular joint. *Journal of Prosthetic Dentistry,* **42**, 191–196

McCloskey, D. I. and Mitchell, J. H. (1972) Reflex cardiovascular and respiratory responses originating in exercising muscle. *Journal of Physiology (London),* **224**, 173–186

McNeil, C. (1983) Craniomandibular (TMJ) disorders – the state of the art. Part II: Accepted diagnostic and treatment modalities. *Journal of Prosthetic Dentistry,* **49**, 393–397

McNeil, C., Danzig, W. M., Farrar, W. B. *et al.* (1980) Craniomandibular (TMJ) disorders – the state of the art. *Journal of Prosthetic Dentistry,* **44**, 434–437

Mejersjö, C. (1984) Long-term development after treatment of mandibular dysfunction and osteoarthrosis. *Swedish Dental Journal*, Suppl. 22

Mejersjö, C. and Carlsson, G. E. (1983) Long-term results of treatment for temporomandibular joint pain-dysfunction. *Journal of Prosthetic Dentistry,* **49**, 809–815

Melzack, R. (1971) Phantom limb pain. *Anaesthesiology,* **35**, 409–419

Melzack, R. (1973) *The Puzzle of Pain*, Penguin Books, New York, pp. 49–60

Mercuri, L. G., Olson, R. E. and Laskin, D. M. (1979) The specificity of response to experimental stress in patients with myofascial pain dysfunction syndrome. *Journal of Dental Research,* **58**, 1866–1871

Møller, E. (1985) Muscle hyperactivity leads to pain and dysfunction. In *Oro-facial Pain and Neuromuscular Dysfunction – Mechanisms and Clinical Correlates* (eds I. Klineberg and B. Sessle), Pergamon, Oxford, Advances in the Biosciences, Vol. 52, pp. 69–92

Møller, E., Rasmussen, O. C. and Bonde-Petersen, F. (1979) Mechanism of ischaemic pain in human muscles of mastication: intramuscular pressure, EMG, force and blood flow of the temporal and masseter muscles during biting. In *Advances in Pain Research and Therapy*, Vol. 3 (eds J. J. Bonica, J. C. Liebeskind and D. G. Albe-Fessard), Raven Press, New York, pp. 271–281

Mohl, N. D., McCall, W. D., Lund, J. P. and Plesh, O. (1990) Devices for the diagnosis and treatment of temporomandibular disorders. Part I: Introduction, scientific evidence, and jaw tracking. *Journal of Prosthetic Dentistry,* **63**, 198–201

Mongini, F., Tempia-Valenta, G. and Benvegnu, G. (1986) Computer-based assessment of habitual mastication. *Journal of Prosthetic Dentistry,* **55**, 638–649

Mongini, F., Ventricelli, F. and Conserva, E. (1988) Etiology of cranio-facial pain and headache in stomatognathic dysfunction. In *Proceedings of the Vth World Congress on Pain* (eds R. Dubner, G. F. Gebhart and M. R. Bond), Elsevier Science Publishers, Amsterdam, pp. 512–519

Montiero, A. A. (1990) *Blood Flow Changes in Human Masseter Muscle Elicited by Voluntary Isometric Contraction*. School of Dentistry, Karolinska Institute, Stockholm, pp. 1–45

Moulton, R. (1955) Oral and dental manifestations of anxiety. *Psychiatry,* **18**, 261–273

Moulton, R. E. (1966) Emotional factors in non-organic temporomandibular joint pain. *Dental Clinics of North America*, 609–620

Moyers, R. E. (1956) Some physiologic considerations of centric and other jaw relations. *Journal of Prosthetic Dentistry,* **6**, 183–194

Munro, A. (1978) Monosynaptic hypochondriacal psychoses. *Canadian Psychiatric Association Journal,* **23**, 497–500

Naeije, M. and Zorn, H. (1981) Changes in the power spectrum of the surface electromyogram of the human masseter muscle due to local muscle fatigue. *Archives of Oral Biology,* **26**, 409–412

Naeije, M. and Hansson, T. L. (1986) Electromyographic screening of myogenous and arthrogenous TMJ dysfunction patients. *Journal of Oral Rehabilitation*, **13**, 433–441

Närhi, M., Byers, M., Hirvonen, T. and Dong, W. (1987) The effect of external irritation on morphology and function of pulpal and dentine nerves. In *Dentine and Dentine Reactions in the Oral Cavity* (eds A. Thylstrup, S. A. Leach and V. Qvist), IRL Press, Oxford, pp. 77–84

Närhi, M. V. O., Hirvonen, T. J. and Hakamäki, M. O. K. (1982) Activation of intradental nerves in the dog to some stimuli applied to the dentine. *Archives of Oral Biology*, **27**, 1053–1058

Nilner, M. (1981) Prevalence of functional disturbances and diseases of the stomatognathic system in 15–18 year olds. *Swedish Dental Journal*, **5**, 189–197

Nilner, M. and Lassing, S.-A. (1981) Prevalence of functional disturbances and diseases of the stomatognathic system in 7–14 year olds. *Swedish Dental Journal*, **5**, 173–187

Ogus, H. D. and Toller, P. A. (1981) *Common Disorders of the Temporomandibular Joint*. John Wright, Bristol, pp. 38–42

Olson, R. E. (1980) Myofascial pain – dysfunction syndrome: psychological aspects. In *The Temporomandibular Joint: A Biological Basis for Clinical Practice* (eds B. G. Sarnat and D. M. Laskin), 3rd edn, C. C. Thomas, Springfield, Ill., pp. 300–314

Olsson, A. (1969) Temporomandibular joint function and functional disturbances. *Dental Clinics of North America*, **13**, 643–665

Peck, C. L. and Kraft, G. H. (1977) Electromyographic biofeedback for pain related to muscle tension. *Archives of Surgery*, **112**, 889–895

Petersson, A. R. (1987) What is an optimal temporomandibular joint radiograph? In *Perspectives in Temporomandibular Disorders* (eds G. T. Clark and W. K. Solberg), Quintessence, Chicago, pp. 59–68

Pilowsky, I. (1978) A general classification of abnormal illness behaviours. *British Journal of Medical Psychiatry*, **51**, 131–137

Posselt, U. (1962) *Physiology of Occlusion and Rehabilitation*, Blackwell Scientific Publications, Oxford, pp. 60–61

Pröschel, P. and Hofmann, M. (1988) Frontal chewing patterns of the incisor point and their dependence on resistance of food and type of occlusion. *Journal of Prosthetic Dentistry*, **59**, 617–624

Ramfjord, S. P. (1961) Bruxism, a clinical and electromyographic study. *Journal of the American Dental Association*, **62**, 22–44

Rasmussen, O. C. (1983) Temporomandibular arthropathy. Clinical, radiologic and therapeutic aspects, with emphasis on diagnosis. *International Journal of Oral Surgery*, **12**, 365–397

Rasmussen, O. C., Bonde-Petersen, F., Christensen, L. V. and Møller, E. (1977) Blood flow in human mandibular elevators at rest and during controlled biting. *Archives of Oral Biology*, **22**, 539–543

Reade, P. C., Burrows, G. D. and Gerschman, J. A. (1977) Oro-facial pain. *Australian Dental Journal*, **22**, 143

Rees, R. T. and Harris, M. (1978) Atypical odontalgia. *British Journal of Oral Biology*, **16**, 212–218

Riise, C. (1983) Clinical and electromyographic studies on occlusion. *Thesis*, Karolinska Institute, Stockholm

Roberts, C. A., Tallens, R. H., Katzberg, R. W. *et al.* (1987a) Clinical and arthrographic evaluation of the location of temporomandibular joint pain. *Oral Surgery*, **64**, 6–8

Roberts, C. A., Tallens, R. H., Katzberg, R. W. *et al.* (1987b) Comparison of arthrographic findings of the temporomandibular joint with palpation of the muscles of mastication. *Oral Surgery*, **64**, 275–277

Rohlin, M., Åkerman, S. and Kopp, S. (1986) Tomography as an aid to detect macroscopic changes of the temporomandibular joint. *Acta Odontologica Scandinavica*, **44**, 131–140

Rosen, H. (1982) Cracked tooth syndrome. *Journal of Prosthetic Dentistry*, **47**, 36–43

Rosenberg, H. M. and Silha, R. E. (1982) TMJ radiography with emphasis on tomography. *Dental Radiography and Photography*, **55**, 1–24

Rugh, J. D. and Solberg, W. K. (1976) Psychological implications in temporomandibular pain and dysfunction. *Oral Sciences Reviews*, **7**, 3–30

Rushton, J., Gibilisco, J. and Goldstein, N. (1959) Atypical face pain. *Journal of the American Medical Association*, **171**, 545–548

Sanchez-Woodworth, R. E., Tallens, R. H., Katzberg, R. W. and Guay, J. A. (1988) Bilateral internal derangements of temporomandibular joint evaluation by magnetic resonance imaging. *Oral Surgery*, **65**, 281–285

Schwartz, G. E. (1975) Biofeedback, self-regulation, and the patterning of physiological processes. *American Scientist*, **63**, 314–324

Schwartz, L. L. (1955) Pain associated with the temporomandibular joint. *Journal of the American Dental Association*, **51**, 394–397

Scott, J. and Humphreys, M. (1987) Psychiatric aspects of dentistry 1. *British Dental Journal*, **163**, 81–88

Sessle, B. J., Hu, J. W., Dubner, R. and Lucier, G. E. (1981) Functional properties in cat trigeminal subnucleus caudalis (medullary dorsal horn) II. Modulation of responses to noxious and non-noxious stimuli by periaqueductal gray, nucleus raphé magnus, cerebral cortex, and afferent influences, and effect of naloxone. *Journal of Neurophysiology*, **45**, 193–207

Sjögaard, G., Savard, G. and Juel, C. (1988) Muscle blood flow during isometric activity and its relation to muscle fatigue. *European Journal of Applied Physiology*, **57**, 327–355

Solberg, W. K. (1979) Temporomandibular and myofascial disorders: Three-part treatment program. In *Proceedings of the Second International Prosthodontic Congress* (ed. W. Lefkowitz), C. V. Mosby, St Louis

Solberg, W. K., Clark, G. T. and Rugh, J. D. (1975) Nocturnal electromyographic evaluation of bruxism patients undergoing short term splint therapy. *Journal of Oral Rehabilitation*, **2**, 215–223

Stahlberg, E. and Eriksson, P. O. (1987) A scanning electromyographic study of the topography of human masseter single motor units. *Archives of Oral Biology*, **32**, 793–797

Sternbach, R. A. (1974) *Pain Patients: Traits and Treatment*, Academic Press, New York

Sumino, R., Nozaki, S. and Katoh, M. (1981) Trigemino-neck reflex. In *Oral-facial Sensory and Motor Functions* (eds Y. Kawamura and R. Dubner), Quintessence, Tokyo, pp. 81–88

Swepston, J. H. and Miller, A. W. (1986) The incompletely fractured tooth. *Journal of Prosthetic Dentistry*, **55**, 413–416

Tallens, R. H., Katzberg, R. W., Miller, T. L. *et al.* (1986) Arthrographically assisted splint therapy: painful clicking with a non-reducing meniscus. *Oral Surgery*, **61**, 2–4

Taylor, A., Elias, S. A. and Somjen, G. (1987) Focal synaptic potentials due to discrete mossy-fibre arrival volleys in the cerebellar cortex. *Proceedings of the Royal Society, London*, **B231**, 217–230

Toller, P. A. (1969) Transpharyngeal radiography for arthritis of the mandibular condyle. *British Journal of Oral Surgery*, **7**, 47–54

Tradowsky, M. and Dworkin, J. B. (1982) Determination of the physiologic equilibrium point of the mandible by electronic means. *Journal of Prosthetic Dentistry*, **48**, 89–98

Travel, J. (1960) Temporomandibular joint pain referred from muscles of the head and neck. *Journal of Prosthetic Dentistry*, **10**, 745–763

Travel, J. and Rinzler, S. H. (1952) The myofascial genesis of pain. *Postgraduate Medicine*, **11**, 425–434

Travel, J. G. and Simons, D. G. (1983) *Myofascial Pain and Dysfunction. The Trigger Point Manual*. Williams & Wilkins, Baltimore, pp. 103–281

Trowbridge, H. O. (1986) Review of dental pain – histology and physiology. *Journal of Endodontics*, **12**, 445–452

Trowbridge, H. O., Franks, M., Korostoff, E. and Emling, R. (1980) Sensory response to thermal stimulation in human teeth. *Journal of Endodontics*, **6**, 405–412

Visser, S. L. and De Rijke, W. (1974) Influence of sex and age on EMG contraction pattern. *European Neurology*, **12**, 229–235

Wallace, C. and Klineberg, I. (1990) Splint therapy for cranio-cervical dysfunction. *Journal of Dental Research*, **69** (Abstr. 21), 935

Wänman, A. (1987) Craniomandibular disorders in adolescents. A longitudinal study in an urgan Swedish population. *Swedish Dental Journal*, Suppl. 44

Wänman, A. and Agerberg, G. (1986a) Mandibular dysfunction in adolescents I. Prevalence of symptoms. *Acta Odontologica Scandinavica*, **44**, 47–54

Wänman, A. and Agerberg, G. (1986b) Mandibular dysfunction in adolescents II. Prevalence of signs. *Acta Odontologica Scandinavica*, **44**, 55–62

Wedel, A. (1988) Heterogeneity of patients with craniomandibular disorders. *Swedish Dental Journal*, Suppl. 55

Wedel, A. and Carlsson, G. E. (1985) Factors influencing the outcome of treatment in patients referred to a temporomandibular joint clinic. *Journal of Prosthetic Dentistry*, **54**, 420–426

Wenneberg, B. (1983) Inflammatory involvement of the temporomandibular joint. *Swedish Dental Journal*, Suppl. 20

Wenneberg, B. and Kopp, S. (1978) Short term effect of intra-articular injections of a corticosteroid on temporomandibular joint pain and dysfunction. *Swedish Dental Journal*, **2**, 189–196

Wenneberg, B., Nystrom, T. and Carlsson, G. E. (1988) Occlusal equilibration and other stomatognathic treatment in patients with mandibular dysfunction and headache. *Journal of Prosthetic Dentistry*, **59**, 478–483

Wilkes, C. H. (1978a) Structural and functional alterations of the temporomandibular joint. *North-west Dentistry*, **57**, 287–294

Wilkes, C. H. (1978b) Arthrography of the temporomandibular joint. *Minnesota Medicine*, **61**, 645–652

Witter, D. J., van Elteren, P. and Käyser, A. F. (1988) Signs and symptoms of mandibular dysfunction in shortened dental arches. *Journal of Oral Rehabilitation*, **15**, 413–420

Witter, D. J., van Elteren, P., Käyser, A. F. and van Rossum, G. M. J. M. (1990) Oral comfort in shortened dental arches. *Journal of Oral Rehabilitation*, **17**, 137–143

Wyke, B. D. (1976) Neurological aspects of the diagnosis and treatment of facial pain. In *Scientific Foundations of Dentistry* (eds B. Cohen and I. Kramer), William Heinemann Books, London, pp. 278–299

Wyke, B. (1977) Neurological aspects of low back pain. In *The Lumbar Spine and Back Pain* (ed M. I. V. Jayson), Sector Publishing, London, pp. 189–256

Yemm, R. (1971) A comparison of the electrical activity of masseter and temporal muscles of human subjects during experimental stress. *Archives of Oral Biology*, **16**, 269–273

Yemm, R. (1979) Neurophysiologic studies of temporomandibular joint dysfunction. In *Temporomandibular Joint Function and Dysfunction* (eds G. A. Zarb and G. E. Carlsson), Munksgaard, Copenhagen, pp. 215–237

Zarb, G. A. and Carlsson, G. E. (1988) Therapeutic concepts: an overview. In *A Textbook of Occlusion* (eds N. D. Mohl, G. A. Zarb, G. E. Carlsson and J. D. Rugh), Quintessence, Chicago, pp. 265–270

Zarb, G. A. and Speck, J. E. (1977) The treatment of temporomandibular joint dysfunction: a retrospective study. *Journal of Prosthetic Dentistry*, **38**, 420–432

Differential diagnosis and management of orofacial pain derived from nerves, vessels and miscellaneous conditions

Table 3.1 Other causes of orofacial pain

NERVES
  Primary neuralgias
    Trigeminal
    Geniculate
    Glossopharyngeal
  Secondary neuralgias
    Post-herpetic neuralgia
    Traumatic neuropathies
    Causalgia
    Auriculotemporal syndrome
VESSELS
  Superficial vascular pain
    Facial migraine
    Temporal arteritis
  Deep vascular pain
    Cranial migraine

3.1 Introduction

Orofacial pain may arise from other structures and tissues and most importantly from nerves and blood vessels (Table 3.1). As a result of the referral of pain to superficial tissues and often over a large area of head and face, the specific features of pain from particular tissues should be understood.

The following information briefly summarizes the characteristic features of pain arising from nerves and vessels, and the section on miscellaneous pains discusses a number of the less commonly occurring pain problems. The clinician must be aware that a variety of causes of orofacial pain exists and that the less common problems nevertheless do occur.

3.2 Nerves

3.2.1 Primary trigeminal neuralgia (tic douloureux)

Trigeminal neuralgia is the more commonly occurring neuralgia, and pain distribution follows the dermatomal innervation of superficial facial tissues. Trigeminal neuralgia may involve the mandibular, maxillary or ophthalmic divisions, with the mandibular division involved most frequently and the ophthalmic branch least frequently.

Neuralgia presents with acutely distressing paroxysmal, lancinating pain, often triggered by light touch of superficial facial tissues; each burst of pain lasts a few seconds and is followed by a short period of reduced pain, followed by a further burst of pain and so on. The overall pain episode lasts several minutes, and there is usually complete remission between attacks.

Lance (1975) describes trigeminal neuralgia in graphic terms which fully captures the distressing features of this type of pain:

> Any pain originating in the trigeminal nerve may properly be called trigeminal neuralgia, and yet the term is usually applied to a particular type of pain, distinctive and devastating, which strikes its victim like lightning. Unlike lightning, it strikes the same place more than once, again and again, until its repeated jabs may drive the patient to despair.

The characteristics of the pain are as follows:

1. It is unilateral (95% cases, unless in the presence of multiple sclerosis (Anthony, 1979).
2. It is triggered by light touch of the skin or slight stretch of the skin or mucous membrane with changes in facial expression;
3. It affects older adults (over 50 years) most commonly, and when present in younger adults suggests the presence of a debilitating systemic disease such as multiple sclerosis (Anthony, 1979; Mitchell, 1980);
4. It involves the mandibular branch of the trigeminal nerve most commonly;
5. It occurs more frequently in women (ratio 2:1);
6. Management of trigeminal neuralgia initially involves the use of the drug carbamazepine (Tegretol).

In fully edentulous patients presenting with paroxysmal pain and where there appears to be a loss of vertical dimension of occlusion, it may be beneficial for a variable time to restore the lost vertical jaw height. This procedure has been successful in managing trigeminal neuralgia in some patients (Lindsay, 1969); however, the mechanism producing the pain must be different from true trigeminal neuralgia. In these cases, the variation in jaw height must affect afferent projections within the brain-stem trigeminal system thereby altering the inhibitory balance of transmission neurones, so as to suppress nociceptive transmission.

True trigeminal neuralgia, however, will not respond to alterations in vertical dimension of occlusion and clearly involves a different mechanism. Possible causes of true trigeminal neuralgia include:

1. Degenerative changes in myelin sheaths surrounding trigeminal nerve branches;
2. Compression of trigeminal ganglion by an atherosclerotic branch of the superior cerebellar artery (Jannetta, 1976; Weidmann, 1979);
3. A structural abnormality related to ageing (Kerr, 1963); or
4. A neurological abnormality (Wyke, 1976; Calvin, Loeser and Howe, 1977).

Pre-trigeminal neuralgia has been described (Mitchell, 1980) where, before the onset of the characteristic symptoms of trigeminal neuralgia, other symptoms may be present for a few days to several years.

The pain is commonly 'burning', or 'aching' and 'burning' varying from mild to severe. The pain episodes are variable in frequency and duration. In general, dull aching, burning pain may occur when provoked by touch or pressure on the face or with drinking hot or cold liquids. Pain occurs in one of the alveolar quadrants and, although there are no significant radiographic features, there may be an association between poor dental health (poor plaque control, active caries present, etc.) and this condition. Differential diagnosis may be difficult but the dull aching, burning pain in an alveolar quadrant without an obvious explanation may be pre-trigeminal neuralgia. Management is with carbamazepine (Tegretol).

Trigeminal neuralgia is often complicated by atypical facial pain – perhaps as a secondary phenomenon. Failure to recognize this may suggest that the trigeminal neuralgia is not responsive to medication and may lead to unnecessary surgery. Management with tricyclic medication in combination with carbamazepine is very effective (Harris, 1991; personal communication).

3.2.2 Secondary trigeminal neuralgia

A variety of peripheral lesions may present with trigeminal neuralgia-like symptoms; conditions of carcinoma of the maxillary antrum, nasopharyngeal carcinoma, benign tumours such as meningiomas, neuromas or fibromas may also present symptoms similar to trigeminal neuralgia pain.

More commonly, secondary neuralgias follow herpes zoster; however, occasionally following herpes simplex (Stalker, 1980), where trauma to peripheral nerves results in the formation of neuropathies at the site of nerve damage. This may lead to causalgia or the auriculotemporal syndrome.

Post-herpetic neuralgia more commonly follows an attack of herpes zoster (or shingles). The virus is the same as that causing chicken pox and post-herpetic neuralgia may follow a reactivation by the virus at a later time. Vesicular eruptions on the skin occur over the distribution of the ophthalmic divisions of the trigeminal nerve in the majority of cases. The area affected may remain numb or aching and pain arises spontaneously without stimulation.

Less commonly the geniculate ganglion may be involved, resulting in a vesicular eruption of the skin in the external ear canal in association with facial palsy involving the seventh cranial nerve (Ramsay-Hunt syndrome). In this case the condition is known as geniculate herpes.

Pain of post-herpetic neuralgia often disturbs sleep and in most cases improves spontaneously within 12–18 months (Anthony, 1979).

3.2.3 Management

Premedication laboratory tests are desirable (Bayer and Stenger, 1979) and should include a blood count, platelet count, reticulocyte count and serum iron analysis, as well as urinalysis. These tests should be repeated at weekly intervals for the first month and then at monthly intervals for 2–3 years.

Carbamazepine (Tegretol) is prescribed in increasing doses beginning with 100 mg t.d.s. and increasing to 300–400 mg t.d.s. until a suitable maintenance level is reached. Unfortunately Tegretol may not be effective long term and other treatments may then be required. These may involve local alcohol injection into the peripheral nerve branch; thermocoagulation of the appropriate division in the trigeminal ganglion using a stereotactic probe (Anthony, 1979); or decompression of the appropriate division (Jannetta, 1976).

3.3 Vessels

Vascular pains in the face are distinct in that their distribution follows the course of facial arteries (not nerves) and the throbbing nature of the pain is distinct from neuralgia pain. Vascular headaches may be provoked by a wide variety of conditions. Table 3.2 lists several possibilities.

3.3.1 Migraine

Migraine may be regarded as a hereditary paroxysmal vasoregulative instability, and comprises episodes in which a phase of intracerebral arterial constriction is followed by a phase of extracerebral arterial dilatation. The precise cause is not known. However, two theories are

Table 3.2 Vascular headaches – possible causes

Systemic lupus erythematosus
Coital headache (BP, low CSF pressure)
Essential hypertension
Altitude headache (hypoxia causing vasodilation of cranial vessels)
Alcohol – 'hangover' (ethanol)
Ice cream headache (cold causing reflex vasospasm)
Food or beverage headache
   Citrus fruit (possible allergy)
   Chocolate, cheese (tryamine, phenylethylamine as trigger factors)
   Dairy products (possible allergy)
   'Hot dog' (sodium nitrite)
   'Chinese restaurant' headache (monosodium glutamate)
   Vitamin A (>50 000 I.U. vitamin A)

suggested to explain the vascular changes that are known to occur through blood flow studies (Anthony, 1983):

1. Sympathetic overactivity (Anthony, 1981, 1983)
    (a) Intracerebral and extracerebral vessels contain adrenergic nerve fibres from the superior cervical ganglia;
    (b) α- and β-adrenoreceptors are found in these arteries and stimulation of α-receptors causes vasoconstriction and stimulation of β-receptors causes vasodilatation;
    (c) β-adrenoreceptors are found in greater density in extracranial rather than intracranial arteries;
    (d) Plasma levels of noradrenaline, dopamine β-hydroxylase and cyclic-AMP increase during migraine attacks and indicate increased sympathetic activity;
    (e) Propranalol, a β-adrenoreceptor antagonist, has been shown to be effective in reducing the frequency and severity of migraine attacks in clinical trials.
2. Serotonin deficiency. A reduction in circulating serotonin as occurs in spontaneous migraine, with a corresponding reduction in vascular tone, is the second possible explanation for the vascular changes. Serotonin normally maintains blood vessel tone, so a reduction in serotonin levels, as occurs during a migraine attack, allows a reduction in blood vessel tone with corresponding vasodilation.

Classic migraine presents with headache associated with premonitory sensory, motor or visual symptoms; *common* migraine describes a condition where there is no focal neurological disturbance preceding the headache and the latter is the more frequent clinical problem.

Management of migraine
1. Simple analgesics such as aspirin or paracetamol are effective in many patients and should be used initially.
2. Ergotamine tartrate is commonly used in the management of migraine. It is an α-adrenoreceptor agonist and constricts the external carotid artery and its branches. It does not have an effect on intracranial arteries.

Table 3.3 Migraine

GENERAL
  Adult incidence F:M–3:1
  (75%F)
  Childhood incidence M>F
  (70%M)
  Age at onset
    2–40 yr (20% < 10 yr)
    20–30 yr (30%)
  Family history (60–70%)
  Response to ergotamine

SYMPTOMS
  Severe, intermittent, throbbing
  Unilateral (50%)
  Nocturnal (not uncommon)
  Present on awakening
  (common)
  Prodromal symptoms (usually
  visual)

ASSOCIATED FEATURES
  Nausea   (90%)
  Vomiting   (60%)
  Photophobia (hypersensitive to
  light)   (80%)
  Visual disturbances
    photopsia (flashing light)
  Light-headedness   (70%)
  Scalp tenderness   (65%)
  Vertigo   (30%)
  Lacrimation
  Mood alteration

3. Auxiliary drugs such as sedatives (5 mg diazepam) or hypnotics (5–10 mg nitrazepam or 500 mg chloral hydrate) may help when used with analgesics or ergotamine tartrate but are addictive.

4. Serotonin inhibitors such as methysergide or pizotifen may also be effective in some patients. Methysergide was the first competitive serotonin antagonist and so competes for receptor sites and is particularly effective when blood levels of serotonin fall. The administration of amitriptyline at night as well, enhances the effectiveness of methysergide. It is important to stop treatment for one month in every five to reduce the risk of the complication of retroperitoneal fibrosis. Pizotifen is not as effective as methysergide but has less side effects and is chemically related to tricyclic antidepressants, which may be beneficial.

5. Tricyclic antidepressants such as nortriptyline are highly effective in many patients as a long-term prophylactic.

6. β-adrenergic blockers, such as propranolol, are competitive inhibitors of β-adrenoreceptors. An aggravating factor of migraine is hypertension and these drugs are antihypertensive agents and are thus recommended for migraine management in patients suffering also from hypertension.

7. Monoamine oxidase inhibitors (MAOIs). The feature of a reduction in plasma serotonin may be countered by administering MAOIs. These drugs inhibit monoamine oxidase activity and encourage the accumulation of monoamines. In this way the reduction of serotonin may be overcome. MAOIs are recommended for those patients who fail to respond to other migraine therapy and who also present with symptoms of depression.

Table 3.3 summarizes the features of migraine, and Table 3.4 lists a selection of medications that have been used in management of migraine headache.

Table 3.4 Migraine medication (a selection of the more commonly prescribed medications)

	Ancillary medication
1 Acute Attack	

1.1 Analgesics (alone or in combination)
  aspirin
  paracetamol } every 4 hours
	Diazepam 5–10 mg

1.2 Ergotamine tartrate 1 or 2 mg 2 hourly (maximum 5–8 mg per week)	Diazepam 5–10 mg
2 Migraine prevention	
2.1 Propranolol 20 mg twice daily increasing to 40 mg twice daily	Ergotamine 2 mg twice daily
2.2 Pizotifen 0.5 mg nocte increasing to 0.5 mg three times daily	
2.3 Phenelzine (MAOI) 15 mg three times daily (effective in 10–15 days)	
2.4 Nortriptyline 10–50 mg nocte	

3.3.2 Periodic migrainous neuralgia or cluster headache

This condition is distinct from migraine. Its aetiology and diagnosis have been poorly understood judging by the wide variety of terms used to describe this condition: sphenopalatine neuralgia, ciliary neuralgia, vidian neuralgia, histamine cephalgia, Horton's syndrome, atypical facial neuralgia, migraine variant, and others.

Although this condition is genetically, biochemically and clinically different from migraine, it is nevertheless a problem associated with facial and cranial arteries.

Cluster headache is distinct from migraine and is seen more commonly in men (80% male incidence) within the age range of 20–50 years. It is now known to have the characteristic presenting features of:

1. Pain in the head and face but centred behind one eye. Pain is severe, paroxysmal, explosive and always affects the same side. Attacks frequently occur in the evening or at night, and may last from minutes to one to two hours; and
2. Pain occurs over a period of days or weeks and then resolves and may not occur for months or years.

Pain is thought to be caused by a sudden release of histamine, as blood levels increase during an attack, and reddening of the skin with an increase in scalp temperature occurs, suggesting vasodilation.

Table 3.5 summarizes the distinctive features of cluster headache, which should be compared with the features of migraine (Table 3.3).

Medication
Ergotamine tartrate suppositories (0.5–1.0 mg nocte) are used for nocturnal attacks. Otherwise, use of nortriptyline (10–50 mg nocte) or pizotifen (0.5 mg nocte) is recommended.

Many of the medications prescribed for vascular pains have side effects which must be understood, and the recommended dose carefully controlled. It is clear also that the responsibility of management of these conditions should be with the patient's medical practitioner (GP or specialist) with whom the dentist should work closely.

Table 3.6 lists medication appropriate for the management of this condition.

3.3.3 Temporal arteritis

Temporal arteritis or giant-cell arteritis is a collagen disorder mainly affecting the temporal artery but may involve other branches of the carotid artery also. Lance (1981) reported that thermograms have shown cold spots in the supra-orbital region at the beginning of an episode and between attacks. Although Doppler studies indicate a fall in blood flow in the supra-orbital and frontal arteries at the start of an attack, other studies have shown an increase in blood flow.

The condition affects elderly patients (over 55 years) and occurs more frequently in women. Clinical features of the disease include severe,

Table 3.5 Cluster headache – periodic migrainous neuralgia

GENERAL
  Male:Female–4:1
  Age:20–50 yr(mean35 yr)
  No family history of migraine

SYMPTOMS
  Paroxysmal, explosive, periorbital
  Unilateral
  Nocturnal (often)
  Cluster cycles (weeks) with pain-free intervals (weeks–months)

ASSOCIATED FEATURES
  Ipsilateral

Lacrimation	(80%)
Nasal stuffiness	(50%)
Hyperaemic eye	(50%)
Facial flushing	(25%)
Horner's syndrome	(25%)
Running nose	(10%)
Alcohol sensitivity	(50%)

Table 3.6 Cluster headache – medication

Ergotamine tartrate
0.5–1.0 mg suppository, nocte
Pizotifen
  0.5 mg nocte increasing to
  0.5 mg three times daily; or
Nortriptyline 10–50 mg at night

throbbing temporal pain and tenderness of the affected arteries. Systemic symptoms are fatigue, weight loss, possibly fever, polymyalgia and generalized synovitis. There is a raised erythrocyte sedimentation rate (ESR) and peripheral leucocytosis. The particular concern in this condition is the possible involvement of the ophthalmic arteries causing infarction of the optic nerve and blindness (Lance and Anthony, 1980).

Haraldson and Mejersjö (1982) reported on two cases where the initial signs and symptoms were those of craniomandibular disorders. Clinical assessment indicated tender TM joints, tenderness of temporal muscles and limited jaw mobility (20–25 mm inter-incisor opening) with deviation to one side. There were additional symptoms that pointed to temporal arteritis including raised temperature, raised ESR, raised white cell count. Temporal artery biopsy confirmed a chronic inflammatory condition of the tissues. Treatment involved cortisone therapy, commencing with 20 mg prednisone three times daily, and progressively reducing the dose over an extended period (six months). This resulted in resolution of all symptoms after one month, but the medication was continued for six months.

3.4 Miscellaneous conditions

3.4.1 Eagle's syndrome

The presence of an elongated styloid process has been considered as the cause of unilateral or bilateral pain in the throat and face. The following information from the literature represents the commonly held dental view that the styloid process is a cause of pain in the throat. However, it is now apparent that pain presenting as throat pain may be either atypical facial pain or glossopharyngeal neuralgia. Medical management with tricyclic antidepressant medication is indicated (nortriptyline 10–20 mg nocte for six weeks and increasing to 25–100 mg if necessary). Surgical intervention, as described by Baddour, McAnear and Tilson (1978), is not appropriate since the presence of the elongated styloid process is an associated finding rather than the cause of the pain.

The styloid process is usually of the order of 25 mm in length according to Eagle (1958). Elongated processes occur in only 4% of the population and of this group only 4% present with symptoms that may be attributed to the styloid process (Eagle, 1958). It consists of a base immediately anterior to the stylomastoid foramen, and a projection of varying length that gives attachment to the stylohyoid and stylomandibular ligaments, as well as the styloglossus, stylohyoid and stylopharyngeous muscles. The stylohyoid ligament extends from the tip of the styloid process and inserts into the lesser cornu of the hyoid bone. It varies in diameter and may become progressively ossified in older patients. The ligament represents the sheath of cartilage of the second pharyngeal arch of the embryo from which the styloid process and hyoid bone are derived.

Baddour, McAnear and Tilson (1978) and Breault (1986) have reported on cases that presented with chronic unilateral orofacial pain that had been present for several years and were unresponsive to a variety of treatment procedures. The symptoms may include TM joint clicking, pain in the ipsilateral ear, pain on jaw opening and head rotation, and pain with swallowing.

Presenting symptoms such as these may indicate a TM joint dysfunction, but lack of response with routine occlusal therapy requires reassessment of the condition. Specific symptoms that may be attributed to an elongated ligament have been identified by Breault (1986) as:

1. Chronic throat pain, that remains after tonsillectomy;
2. Sensation of a foreign body in the throat;
3. Difficulty in swallowing;
4. Ear pain;
5. Pain along the distribution of the external and internal carotid arteries;
6. Head pain.

Assessment

Radiographic assessment with a screening OPG will show an elongated styloid process, and an anteroposterior projection of the skull will show TM joints and styloid process also. Intra-oral examination is carried out with palpation lateral to the tonsillar fossa, where a bony protuberance may be felt, and this may also cause pain similar to that originally described by the patient. The styloid process lies between the carotid arteries and it is considered that an elongated process may impinge on the internal or external carotid and may diminish vessel diameter and irritate the sympathetic plexus surrounding the artery. Symptoms of pain evoked on head rotation and pain in the cervical triangle area may be due to this. Also, pain on palpation may cause headache over the carotid distribution (Eagle, 1958).

3.4.2 Pterygoid hamulus syndrome

The pterygoid hamulus is a bony process found bilaterally as the posteroinferior extension of the medial pterygoid plate. It is located distomedial to the maxillary tuberosity and varies greatly in size. The process is associated with the function of the tensor palati muscles that tense the soft palate and often the eustachian tube during swallowing and speech.

The tensor palati muscle is the tensor of the soft palate and arises from the spine of the sphenoid bone and the floor of the scaphoid fossa. Its fibres converge on the lower pterygoid plate ending in a fine tendon that runs over the hamular notch at the root of the pterygoid hamulus and into the fibrous aponeurosis of the soft palate. Contraction of the tensor palati tenses the soft palate so that contraction of other muscles may elevate it without distortion. A synovial bursa facilitates the movement of the tendon over the hamulus. The tensor palati is innervated by the mandibular branch of the trigeminal nerve via the otic ganglion. Hypertrophy of the hamulus may affect the function of the tensor palati muscle (Hjørting-Hansen and Lous, 1987).

The pterygoid hamulus may be readily palpated by moving the index finger from the hard palate at the level of the maxillary tuberosity and onto the soft palate. The hamulus is usually identified as a prominence covered by a thin layer of mucous membrane and may be traumatized during mastication, swallowing, tongue pressure or palpation.

Assessment
Symptoms of pterygoid hamulus syndrome include pain in the palate and throat particularly during swallowing and speech, as a result of traumatic irritation. The pain may radiate to the palate, maxilla, and zygomatic area and there may be associated headache. There may also be a minor loss of hearing, pain in the ear, tinnitus and vertigo (Wooten, Tarsitano and Reavis, 1970).

Clinical signs may be hypertrophy and inflammatory hyperaemia of the soft tissues overlying the pterygoid hamulus, and there is likely to be local tenderness on palpation. Differential diagnosis may be confirmed by a local anaesthetic block of the ipsilateral posterior palatine nerve. Hjørting-Hansen and Lous (1987) report that in their experience the incidence is as high as 12%.

Management of the condition requires surgical excision of the hypertrophied section of the hamulus (Hertz, 1964; Wooten, Tarsitano and Reavis, 1970; Hjørting-Hansen and Lous, 1987) with complete resolution of symptoms.

3.4.3 Cervicolingual syndrome

This is a condition in which there is unilateral pain felt in the occipital region of the head that radiates towards the ear and TM joint. There may be a prickling and burning sensation of the skin overlying the area behind the ear, together with numbness of the ipsilateral side of tongue and lack of postural sensation in the cervical spine with instability of the head (Lance and Anthony, 1980; Lous, 1987).

Bertoft and Westerberg (1985) suggest that the condition is related to cervical spondylitis and hypermobility. It is often provoked by sudden head movement.

Assessment
Diagnosis is based on the presenting signs and symptoms.

Management
Avoid sudden head movements and extreme mandibular movements. Occlusal therapy is indicated in the form of resistance (isokinetic) exercises for the jaw. Mobilization exercises with the assistance of a physiotherapist are also indicated.

3.4.4 Alveolar cavitational osteopathosis

Cavitational osteopathosis in alveolar bone has been considered a significant and important cause of atypical facial pain and atypical neuralgias in craniofacial structures (Ratner *et al.*, 1979, 1986; Roberts *et al.*, 1984).

Bone cavities are usually related to:

1. Sites of previous tooth extractions that are not usually visible on radiographs; and
2. Tooth, periodontal and maxillary sinus tissues.

Clinically, the symptoms may vary from dental sensitivity to acute pain triggered by touch of the face, neck, head, and possibly involving arms, legs, back; there may be associated blurred vision, nasal congestion and problems of postural balance (Ratner, Langer and Evins, 1986).

Diagnosis is made on the basis of the presence of a chronic pain problem, with acute episodes that are unresponsive to conventional treatment methods. Intra- and extra-oral palpation of the suspected trigger area may elicit pain, and if so is followed by local anaesthetic infiltration through the mucous membrane and against or into the underlying bone. Local anaesthesia will abolish the pain and trigger areas if there is an underlying area of pathology and cavitation.

Management requires the area to be surgically exposed and for necrotic or soft friable bone with inflammatory tissue to be curetted. The site is irrigated, an antibiotic pack is placed at the site if the lesion is large, or an antibiotic irrigation used if the area is small.

The microbacterial flora of such lesions have been investigated by Socransky *et al.* (1976) who identified a variable, mixed bacterial population of both aerobic and anaerobic microorganisms. Following initial treatment there should be a progressive improvement in severity, duration and frequency of the pain episodes.

This condition may provide an explanation for the chronicity of some pain problems that do not respond to other more routine treatment methods. It should be considered, and careful clinical assessment carried out in the search for a physical cause of chronic pain of craniomandibular origin.

3.4.5 Tardive dyskinesia

Tardive dyskinesia is a drug-induced disorder of motor control commonly involving lips, jaw muscles and tongue. It may cause orofacial pain. This is not a common cause of orofacial pain but may present initially to the dentist because of associated difficulties, such as managing complete dentures.

A careful medical history will provide diagnostic information, as patients suffering from this condition will have a history of long-term medication for a variety of psychiatric disorders (schizophrenia or other psychoses) requiring antipsychotic or tranquillizer drugs.

Medications that may be associated with this condition are (Bassett, Remick and Blasberg, 1986):

chlorpromazine – Largactil
haloperidol – Haldol
thioridazine – Melleril
trifluoperazine – Stelazine

Such medications are prescribed for a variety of conditions including anxiety, dementia, depression and personality disorders.

Clinical signs may include 'worm-like' movements of the tongue initially, later developing into involuntary movements of the tongue inside the mouth and protruding from it grimacing movements of the mouth, as well as puckering, sucking, and smacking movements of the lips (Bassett, Remick and Blasberg, 1986; Thomas, 1988). Orofacial pain may arise in association with trauma of soft tissue, particularly from a removable denture. Management requires discontinuing the medication when the condition is likely to be completely reversible. If this is the case, then dental treatment and improved control of complete dentures is possible. If this is not entirely effective, altering the medication is necessary in consultation with the medical specialist.

References

Anthony, M. (1979) Relief of facial pain. *Current Therapeutics*, **20**, 65–77

Anthony, M. (1981) Biochemical indices of sympathetic activity in migraine. *Cephalgia*, **1**, 83–89

Anthony, M. (1983) Drugs in migraine. *Current Therapeutics*, **24**, 89–113

Baddour, H. M., McAnear, J. T. and Tilson, H. B. (1978) Eagle's syndrome. *Oral Surgery*, **46**, 486–494

Bassett, A., Remick, R. A. and Blasberg, B. (1986) Tardive dyskinesia: an unrecognized cause of orofacial pain. *Oral Surgery*, **61**, 570–572

Bayer, D. B. and Stenger, T. G. (1979) Trigeminal neuralgia: an overview. *Oral Surgery*, **48**, 393–399

Bertoft, E. S. and Westerberg, C.-E. (1985) Further observations on the neck-tongue syndrome. In (Olesch, J., Tfelt-Hahsch, P. and Jehsch, K. eds) *Headache: Proceedings of the Second International Headache Congress*, Copenhagen June 18–21, Cephalgia: Vol. 5, Suppl. 3

Breault, M. R. (1986) Eagle's syndrome: Review of literature and implications in craniomandibular disorders. *Journal of Craniomandibular Practice*, **4**, 324–337

Calvin, W. H., Loeser, J. D. and Howe, J. F. (1977) A neurophysiological theory for the pain mechanism of tic douloureux. *Pain*, **3**, 147–154

Eagle, W. (1958) Elongated styloid process. *Archives of Otolaryngology*, **67**, 172–176

Haraldson, T. and Mejersjö, C. (1982) Temporal arteritis: a report on two cases. *Swedish Dental Journal*, **6**, 121–125

Hertz, R. S. (1964) Pain resulting from elongated pterygoid hamulus: report of case. *Journal of Oral Surgery*, **26**, 209–210

Hjørting-Hansen, E. and Lous, I. (1987) The hamulus-pterygoid syndrome. *Ugeskrift for Laeger*, **149**, 979–982

Jannetta, P. J. (1976) Microsurgical approach to the trigeminal nerve for tic douloureux. *Progress in Neurological Surgery*, **7**, 180–200

Kerr, F. W. L. (1963) The etiology of trigeminal neuralgia. *Archives of Neurology*, **8**, 15–25

Lance, J. W. (1975) *Headache*. Charles Scribner's Sons, New York, p. 33

Lance, J. W. (1981) Headache. *Annals of Neurology*, **10**, 1–10

Lance, J. W. and Anthony, M. (1980) Neck-tongue syndrome on sudden turning of head. *Journal of Neurology, Neurosurgery and Psychiatry*, **43**, 97–101

Lindsay, B. (1969) Trigeminal neuralgia: a new approach. *Medical Journal of Australia*, **56**, 8–13

Lous, I. (1987) The cervicolingual syndrome. *Manual Medicine*, **3**, 63–66

Mitchell, R. G. (1980) Pre-trigeminal neuralgia. *British Dental Journal*, **149**, 167–170

Ratner, E. J., Langer, B. and Evins, M. L. (1986) Alveolar cavitational osteoporosis – manifestations of an infectious process and its implication in the causation of chronic pain. *Journal of Periodontology*, **57**, 593–603

Ratner, E. J., Person, P., Kleinman, D. J. *et al.* (1979) Jaw bone cavities and trigeminal and atypical neuralgias. *Oral Surgery,* **48**, 3–20

Roberts, A. M., Person, P., Chandran, N. B. and Hori, J. M. (1984) Further observations on dental parameters of trigeminal and atypical facial neuralgias. *Oral Surgery,* **58**, 121–129

Socransky, S. S., Stone, C., Ratner, E. J. and Person, P. (1976) Oral pathology and trigeminal neuralgia III. *Journal of Dental Research,* **55** (Special Issue B), 952

Stalker, W. H. (1980) Facial neuralgia associated with recurrent herpes simplex. *Oral Medicine,* **49**, 502–503

Thomas, G. A. (1988) Abnormal movements of the oral-facial region – diagnosis, assessment and control. A guide for the dental clinician. *Australian Prosthodontic Journal,* **2**, 41–45

Weidmann, M. J. (1979) Trigeminal neuralgia – surgical treatment by microvascular decompression of the trigeminal nerve root. *Medical Journal of Australia,* **2**, 628–630

Wooten, J. W., Tarsitano, J. J. and Reavis, D. K. (1970) The pterygoid hamulus: a possible source for swelling, erythema and pain: report of three cases. *Journal of the American Dental Association,* **81**, 688–690

Wyke, B. D. (1976) Neurological aspects of the diagnosis and treatment of facial pain. In *Scientific Foundations of Dentistry* (eds B. Cohen and I. Kramer), William Heinemann, London, pp. 278–299

Additional reading

Lance, J. W. (1982) *Mechanism of Headache*, 4th edn, Butterworth Scientific, London

Raskin, N. H. and Appenzeller, O. (1980) *Headache*. Vol. 14, Series: *Major Problems in Internal Medicine*, W. B. Saunders, Philadelphia

Chapter 4

Occlusal splint therapy

4.1 Introduction

4.2 Construction of occlusal splints

4.3 Fitting occlusal splints

4.4 Management of occlusal splints

4.5 Therapeutic effects of occlusal splints
4.5.1 Psychological
4.5.2 Physiological

4.6 Occlusal splints and general muscle performance

4.7 TM joint unloading and anterior repositioning appliances
4.7.1 Unloading appliances
4.7.2 Repositioning appliances

4.8 Use and care of occlusal splints

References

4.1 Introduction

Occlusal splints are essentially diagnostic appliances (Table 4.1) that are worn short term. However, in cases of chronic parafunction they may be used for long-term management, particularly with nocturnal parafunction where the splint is worn at night only. The advantage of a correctly designed occlusal splint is that with short-term use there are no irreversible effects on jaw muscles, TM joints or teeth. Different types of occlusal splints have been described for different purposes (Hawley, 1919; Krogh-Poulsen, 1969; Farrar, 1972; Timm and Ash, 1977); however, in general, the full-arch flat-plane splint has the most widespread application in management of the occlusion.

Table 4.1 Functions of occlusal splints

1. To provide the possibility for spatial change in jaw position to a more harmonious jaw relationship with respect to TM joints and jaw muscles
2. To allow jaw muscles to re-establish a coordinated pattern of activity in the absence of the influence of tooth guidance
3. To encourage appropriate condyle-interarticular disc function when muscle dysfunction is the cause of the dysfunction and/or pain
4. To allow manual jaw guidance to be carried out more easily and so provide the opportunity for jaw registration to be made more accurately
5. To allow resolution of the effects of microtrauma on muscle (which may involve muscle fibre or connective tissue elements or both) leading to inflammation, oedema, pain and an alteration in coordinated muscle activity designed to protect the damaged muscle or region within it

The full-arch splint is designed to cover all of either the maxillary or mandibular teeth, and to provide flat-plane contact against the opposing tooth cusps. Ash and Ramfjord (1982) recommend a maxillary splint. The splint should incorporate the following design features:

1. Flat plane contact with opposing cusp tips at retruded jaw position (RP) to provide bilateral simultaneous contacts on posterior teeth;
2. Guidance on anterior teeth for lateral and protrusive jaw movements; and
3. Bilateral simultaneous contacts around the arch on anterior and posterior teeth at median occlusal position (MOP) (McNamara, 1976, 1978).

This will provide enhanced jaw support at tooth contact and allow smooth lateral and protrusive movements for fluent jaw muscle function. Following adjustments of the appliance at RP, the condyles will adopt an optimal position in their fossae according to the contour of the bone and interarticular discs, and the splint may then be used long term without detrimental effect. Indeed, when used for patients with jaw muscle dysfunction, the occlusal splint may allow resolution of the effects of muscle microtrauma and associated symptoms of pain and/or discomfort. The splint prevents tooth guidance from influencing jaw muscle function, thus allowing reorganization of jaw muscle coordination to protect the painful site and to assist the resolution of pain and dysfunction. It should be emphasized that occlusal splints will have such beneficial effects when dysfunction or pain is directly associated with jaw muscles or joints and where tooth guidance appears to be involved in the aetiology of the dysfunction. After correct fitting and support, follow-up examination is necessary; if there is no change in symptoms two to four weeks later, the case must be reassessed.

It is desirable for occlusal splints to be prepared on articulated study casts with careful waxing to the correct specifications (Table 4.2) for each case (which also minimizes clinical adjustment time) and processed in clear heat-cured acrylic resin (Timm and Ash, 1977; Ash and Ramfjord, 1982; Klineberg, 1983).

Table 4.2 Specifications of occlusal splints

1. To disclude teeth by flat-plane contact against opposing cusp tips
2. To provide bilaterally balanced jaw support at retruded and median occlusal positions
3. To provide freedom for jaw movements from retruded and median occlusal positions
4. To provide anterior guidance for lateral and protrusive jaw movements

Alternatively, a polyurethane appliance that is vacuum moulded and worn as a mouth guard for 'contact' sports is an entirely different appliance. In this instance there is no provision for improved jaw support at RP, and the customary uniform thickness of the appliance from the molar to the incisor region causes bilateral distraction of TM joint condyles with clenching and may encourage interarticular disc displacement. This type of appliance should not be worn long term, as it may also allow changes in tooth alignment to occur.

A combination of hard acrylic base and a soft acrylic surface for occlusal contact has been described (Heir, Berrett and Worth, 1983) cushioning the occlusal contacts in order to reduce their effects on acutely inflamed TM joints.

4.2 Construction of occlusal splints

1. The splint is constructed in clear heat-cured acrylic resin that covers the lingual and occlusal surfaces of the teeth and 2–3 mm of the labial and buccal surfaces. The labial and buccal coverage should be sufficient to prevent tooth movement and provide adequate retention. The lingual coverage increases flexional resistance (Figures 4.1, 4.2).
2. The splint may be constructed for either the maxillary or mandibular arch, depending on the jaw relationship. A maxillary splint most readily allows contact with appropriate opposing tooth cusps, provides anterior guidance, and is preferred for these reasons, although a maxillary splint will interfere with speech more noticeably for the first week of use until the neuromuscular system adapts to its presence.

Figure 4.1 Occlusal splint – waxed form.

(a) Palatal outline of splint on maxillary cast.

(b) Buccal view of the degree of overlap on buccal and labial tooth surfaces; with maxillary and mandibular casts separated by 1.0 mm in the molar region.

(c) Labial view of splint form in wax showing flat-plane contact with mandibular incisor teeth.

(d) Buccal view of splint form in wax showing flat-planed contact with mandibular posterior tooth cusps.

(e) Labial view of splint form in wax to show canine elevation in left laterotrusion. NOTE: only slight contour change is necessary.

(f) Buccal view of splint form in wax to show canine elevation and disclusion of posterior teeth.

(From Klineberg, 1983)

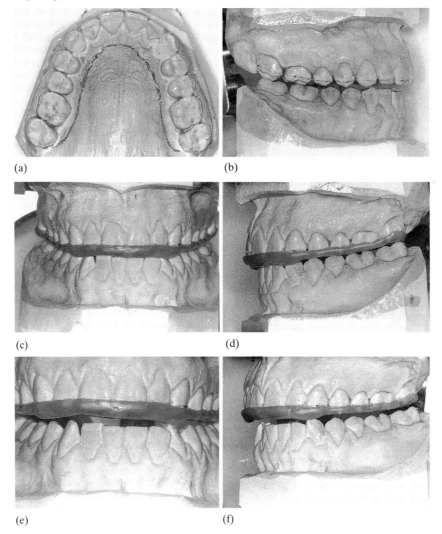

(a)　　　　　　　　　　(b)

(c)　　　　　　　　　　(d)

(e)　　　　　　　　　　(f)

3. The occlusal surface is flat except for two inclined planes placed labial to the canine teeth (Figures 4.1, 4.2). It is not necessary for all cusps on opposing teeth to contact the flat surface in MOP or RP closure for short-term use if this causes the surface of the splint to be too irregular. However, for long-term use, supporting cusps on all opposing teeth should contact the splint surface.

4. The buccolingual contacting surface of the splint is determined by the orientation of the long axis of the lower posterior teeth. If the mandibular molars are tilted lingually, the splint should not be extended below the occlusal plane in order to make contact with lingual cusps, since, if this was done, a very steep canine guidance would be needed to avoid mediotrusive interferences on the splint.

5. Occlusal forces should be directed axially so that anterior contact is determined by the orientation of the long axis of the mandibular anterior teeth (Figure 4.2).

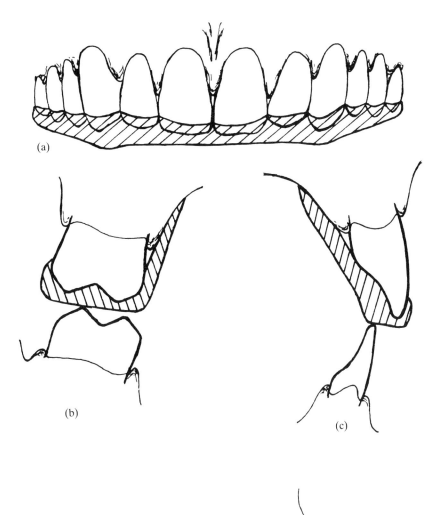

Figure 4.2 Occlusal splint – outline form.

(a) Diagrammatic representation of the outline of a maxillary occlusal splint to illustrate labial and buccal overlap for retention.

(b) and (c) Diagrammatic representation of the contact of mandibular molar cusp and mandibular incisor tooth, against opposing surface of a maxillary occlusal splint. Note lingual and palatal extension of splint.

(d) Diagrammatic representation of the contact of the mandibular teeth against the flat opposing surface of a maxillary occlusal splint. Note buccal and labial overlap and smooth elevation in region of maxillary canine to provide canine guidance. (From Klineberg, 1983)

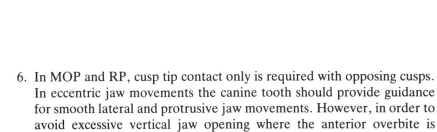

6. In MOP and RP, cusp tip contact only is required with opposing cusps. In eccentric jaw movements the canine tooth should provide guidance for smooth lateral and protrusive jaw movements. However, in order to avoid excessive vertical jaw opening where the anterior overbite is deep, it may be necessary to have canine and incisor guidance in protrusion.

7. Casts are accurately mounted in RP on an articulator and are aligned for splint waxing by adjusting the incisal pin so that a minimum of 1.0 mm separates the closest contacting tooth surfaces (usually the molar lingual cusp tips); this ensures that at its thinnest point the splint is at least 1.0 mm thick. Lateral recordings are made to set condylar guidances of the articulator and the incisal guidance is set with respect to the natural anterior tooth arrangement (Figure 4.1).

8. An outline of the splint is made on the maxillary cast in pencil and baseplate wax is added to provide the appropriate coverage and contour (Figure 4.1). Where interproximal or gingival undercuts are present, it may be necessary to block out these undercuts before beginning the waxing procedure. This may be done with plaster on the working cast (Timm and Ash, 1977; Ash and Ramfjord, 1982) or prepared in wax on a master cast which is then duplicated.

4.3 Fitting occlusal splints

The occlusal splint should be carefully fitted so that it is well retained by the supporting teeth. The labial and buccal overlap provides retention (Figure 4.1), since polymerization shrinkage of the acrylic resin is directed towards the centre of the appliance. Once it is stable against the teeth, jaw support is examined and adjusted using GHM tape* supported by Miller† holders (Figure 4.3).

RP contacts are examined first by guiding the jaw along the terminal hinge arc of closure. Contact markings are adjusted until an even bilateral distribution of stops is apparent in bicuspid and molar areas (Figure 4.3). MOP stops may then be examined and adjusted using a different coloured tape by having the patient snap the jaw closed from an open position in the absence of manual guidance. MOP contacts approximate functional contacts and are usually slightly anterior to RP stops. The splint is then adjusted to provide an even distribution of MOP stops without removing RP stops. Lateral and protrusive movements are finally examined with manual guidance. Eccentric contacts on the splints should occur on the canine elevations or in the canine and incisor regions (Table 4.2). The splint surface is finally polished for patient comfort.

Following fitting of the splint certain problems may present to the patient and are caused by the sudden increase in vertical dimension of occlusion, since splint thickness is of the order of 3 mm anteriorly and 1 mm posteriorly. These effects are:

1. A heightened sensory awareness of teeth and mouth due to pressure stimulation of mucosal receptors of palate and tongue, and a splinting effect of supporting teeth, altering the customary tooth movement within the periodontal space and thus the afferent information from periodontal receptors;

*Gebr. Hanel-Medizinal, D7440 Nürtingen, Germany.
†Gebr. Martin, D7200 Tuttlingen, Germany.

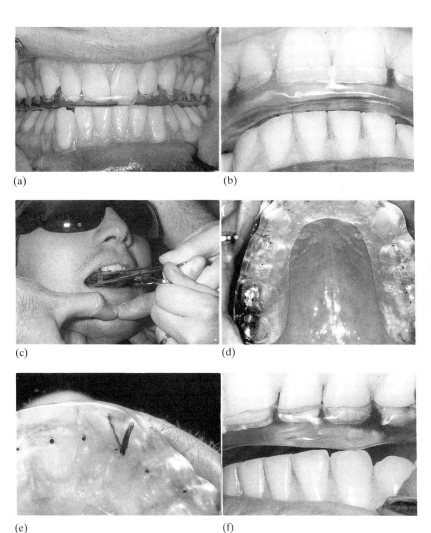

Figure 4.3 Occlusal splint – clinical aspects.

(a) Maxillary occlusal splint in position showing flat-plane contact with opposing mandibular teeth and minimal canine elevation for lateral guidance.

(b) Anterior region of maxillary occlusal splint showing labial overlap for retention and contact with mandibular anterior teeth.

(c) Operator carrying out bilateral guidance of patient's jaw for assessment of retruded position contacts on the splint. Assistant supports GHM tape in Miller holders.

(d) Palatal view of maxillary occlusal splint in position showing outline and extent of palatal coverage and distribution of MOP stops (more anterior and lighter) and RP stops (more posterior and darker). RP stops may be present in the bicuspid and molar area only, but in this case both RP and MOP stops are present around the arch.

(e) Maxillary splint in region of canine elevation to show protrusive (more anterior) and lateral (more posterior) guidance paths marked with GHM tape.

(f) Maxillary splint in region of canine elevation to show lower canine passing along the canine rise in a lateral movement from RP and resulting in disclusion of posterior teeth (see also Figures 4.1, (e) and (f). ((c), (d), (e), (f) from Klineberg, 1983)

2. A reduction of interocclusal space and speaking space;
3. A reduced tongue space initially due to splint thickness;
4. Speech difficulty; and
5. Chewing difficulty, although it is customary for the splint to be removed at meal times. See end of this Chapter for patient instruction information.

4.4 Management of occlusal splints

It is desirable for the splint to be worn during the day (if the patient is prepared to do this) and at night, in order for therapeutic effects to be achieved more quickly. However, particular occupations may cause difficulties for daytime use of the splint, especially if they require predominantly face to face contact and/or speaking (e.g. teachers, receptionists, telephonists, secretaries, sales people etc.).

It is desirable for occlusal splints to be examined and adjusted within seven days of initial fitting and at weekly intervals until jaw support is stable, as indicated by GHM tape markings. At adjustment appointments, similar assessment of splint to opposing tooth contact is made at RP and MOP using GHM tape. At the conclusion of each such appointment, jaw support is balanced, i.e. there are bilateral stops over the bicuspid and molar regions at RP, and a bilateral distribution of stops at MOP that may also involve anterior teeth, since there is no manual guidance required for recording MOP.

Adjustment appointments should continue until there is no observed alteration in opposing tooth stops on the splint on two consecutive appointments. Progressive adjustments are needed whilst jaw muscle coordination changes. The presence of the splint between opposing teeth prevents natural tooth contact, thus a reprogramming of jaw muscles occurs to the new vertical dimension of occlusion defined by the splint. The alteration in jaw muscle activity allows the jaw and TM joints to adopt an optimal spatial position; however, this will not be fully achieved without progressive adjustments. The reorientation of the jaw that occurs in the absence of tooth guidance emphasizes the important influence that tooth arrangement and contact pattern has upon mastication, swallowing and jaw posture.

Progressive changes in jaw support caused by tooth loss, tilting and drifting of unsupported teeth, under-contoured restorations, tooth re-alignments etc., will result in changes in the coordinated activity of jaw muscles (Lous, Sheikholeslam and Møller, 1970; Troelstrup and Møller, 1970; Ingervall and Carlsson, 1982), in the timing of the individual muscle contractions, and in the relative amplitudes of activity. Should the degree of jaw displacement at tooth contact cause sufficient reflex muscle changes, this may contribute to muscle pain and joint dysfunction.

Following the use of an occlusal splint for two to four weeks, a number of changes in jaw position and jaw muscles may occur:

1. The re-establishment of interocclusal space as a result of a change in jaw posture evoked by the increased vertical dimension of occlusion, resulting in an increase in postural muscle length by the acquisition of additional sarcomeres in series (Goldspink, 1976);
2. Resolution of speech difficulty in most patients, although this may not occur fully where a deep incisor overbite is present;
3. Enhanced airway maintenance associated with changes in tongue posture and muscle coordination, with changes in postural jaw position;
4. Resolution of muscle spasm and/or reflex muscle hyperactivity (Yemm, 1979); and
5. Resolution of muscle pain (if the pain problem was caused by progressive alteration in tooth contacts and jaw support, resulting in an unstable re-alignment of the jaw in conjunction with reflex changes in jaw muscle coordination).

4.5 Therapeutic effects of occlusal splints

4.5.1 Psychological effects

Any appliance placed in the mouth will have a psychophysiological effect due to the psychological importance of the mouth over a broad range of sensorimotor functions and because of the profuse sensory innervation of orofacial tissues. However, a correctly designed and adjusted occlusal splint will also provide improved jaw support, and allow spatial re-orientation of the jaw into an optimal position as a result of reprogramming of jaw muscles in the absence of tooth guidance; such guidance being the most important constraint for jaw muscle function (Gibbs *et al.*, 1971; Gibbs *et al.*, 1981; Klineberg, 1980). These effects will result in a subjective feeling of increased comfort with biting, thus allowing a relative increase in bite force in some individuals.

Where the individual has subjective (symptoms) or objective (signs) evidence of jaw muscle dysfunction, the sensorimotor change following splint therapy may be more noticeable, as it may allow a resolution of signs and/or symptoms. Also, a placebo response may be expected, especially if the fitting of the appliance is accompanied by strong and positive suggestions concerning its potential therapeutic value. Thus, in general, there will be a favourable response from the patient concerning comfort of both jaw position and biting.

4.5.2 Physiological effects

From a physiological view point it is known that the tension developed by a muscle varies with its length. Above and below the optimum sarcomere length, muscle tension, and thus the force exerted by the muscle, decreases. The optimal length differs for each muscle and coincides with the length at which the muscle normally functions. With jaw muscles, maximal force is developed at several millimetres of jaw opening rather than at intercuspal position (IP) (Nordström and Yemm, 1972, 1974). Different jaw muscles develop their maximal twitch tensions (or force) at different degrees of jaw opening (Thexton and Hiiemae, 1975) as indicated in the case of the temporal muscle which develops maximal twitch tension at a wide open position; the masseter muscle maximum occurs at a more closed jaw position and the medial pterygoid muscle develops its maximum force closer to IP.

Thus, the placement of an occlusal splint provides an increase in contact vertical dimension of the order of 3 mm at the incisors and 1 mm at the molars and will allow the development of an increased bite force. The degree of bite force possible in an individual varies with the morphology of the facial skeleton, so that greater bite force may be expected where there is a small gonial angle and a relatively large mandibular body, and where there is a strong tendency for the occlusal plane and base bone of the upper and lower jaws to be parallel (Møller, 1966; Ringqvist, 1973; Ingervall and Thilander, 1974).

The use of a correctly designed occlusal splint allowing re-orientation of the jaw may also have an effect on cervical and upper limb musculature.

This is often apparent in the management of pain-dysfunction problems (Wallace and Klineberg, 1990) where there are associated neck and shoulder symptoms.

This occurs because of the close association of trigeminal and cervical nerves, due to the continuity of the spinal nucleus of the trigeminal nerve and the nucleus caudalis of the spinal cord. The former is the principal centre for subserving nociceptive sensations in the head, and this continuity at C2–C4 level provides intimate associations with afferents of upper cervical spinal nerves. As well as trigeminal afferents, facial, hypoglossal and vagal cranial nerve afferents pass through the spinal tract and provide branches to the spinal nucleus, especially in the caudal region.

There are also close associations between cranial motor nuclei and upper cervical motor nuclei. Thus the convergence of upper cervical, trigeminal and other cranial nerve afferents allows complex sensory and motor intercommunications with excitatory and inhibitory influences providing mutual modulation of trigeminal and cervical sensory and motor functions.

4.6 Occlusal splints and general muscle performance

A number of claims (Eversaul, 1977; Jakush, 1982) have been made concerning the use of a variety of different types of occlusal splints – heat-processed acrylic resin maxillary or mandibular occlusal splints, flexible mouth guards, vacuum-formed interocclusal appliances, and mandibular orthopaedic repositioning appliances (MORAs) (Gelb, 1977) and the resulting enhancement of general muscle performance.

This subject has aroused considerable interest because of the possible potentiating effect produced by occlusal appliances on total muscle performance in sport. Claims of an improvement in sporting ability following use of occlusal splints, however, have been largely subjective, although it is clear from the foregoing (see therapeutic effects of an occlusal splint, Section 4.5) that the use of particular appliances can be of considerable benefit to the individual. These general sensorimotor benefits appear to have been responsible for claims by some clinicians of wide ranging improvements in athletic performance of their patients. Clinical studies with control groups for certain sports have suggested that these claims are placebo responses only, there being no improvement in general muscle performance when objectively quantified (Greenberg *et al.*, 1981).

However, weight lifting may be one sport where individual performance is enhanced by use of occlusal splints. This sport requires synchronous coordination of all trunk and limb musculature at maximal isometric contractions for maximal lifting. It is conceivable that in wearing an occlusal splint, the improved jaw comfort and bite force may allow short-term gains in maximum contractions of related muscle groups (particularly neck and shoulder muscles) which could be beneficial for overall performance. However, this situation is totally different from most other sports where transient sequential coordinated bursts of muscle activity are required (rather than synchronous coordination) and usually without tooth contact or jaw muscle clenching.

4.7 TM joint unloading and anterior repositioning appliances

Another type of occlusal appliance may be indicated in the presence of intra-articular derangements of the TM joints. The conditions of reciprocal clicking (Farrar, 1972), closed-lock (Wilkes, 1978) and crepitus may present alone or with pain and may be treated conservatively in many cases. However, the standard occlusal splint just described that is designed with reference to the terminal hinge axis of the TM joints may not be appropriate, although it may be fitted initially where painful crepitus is present.

Clinical management of closed-lock (and sometimes crepitus with pain, especially when associated with an acute arthritic episode), requires unloading of the affected TM joint(s). Reciprocal clicking, especially when associated with pain, requires re-alignment of the condyles downwards and forwards, together with a forward positioning of the mandibular body and dental arch.

The degree of jaw and condyle re-alignment may be assessed with:

1. Standardized transcranial radiographs of TM joints to show the spatial position of condyles and fossae, or;
2. Use of the resiliency test (Palla, 1979) to assess the degree of articular compressibility or vertical condylar displacement.

4.7.1 Unloading appliances (Figures 4.4, 4.5)

An articulator is required that is designed to provide vertical and anteroposterior adjustments of the condylar elements (Klineberg, 1983). The Condylator* is the only articulator currently available with a vernier adjustment for condylar element re-alignment. The Denar† Mark II with option A has an IP–RP (CO–CR) adjustment that allows anteroposterior repositioning, and its arcon design allows the use of shim inserts placed against the superior wall of the fossa box, for vertical re-alignment of the condylar spheres. Such adjustments may be made on the articulator to provide the necessary re-alignment of the articulated casts. The required adjustments of the articulator may be assessed with the aid of standardized transcranial TM joint radiographs that are a guide to the spatial position of the TM condyles. The articulator adjustment of the condylar sphere is made to the extent indicated on the radiographs. The alternative resilience test allows an assessment of the vertical compressibility of the TM joints and interarticular disc, as a guide to appropriate articulator adjustment.

The articulator re-alignment often requires an anteroposterior repositioning of the lower cast of the order of 2–3 mm, and distraction of the condylar spheres of the order of 1 mm (Figure 4.4). The re-alignment allows an unloading and anterior repositioning appliance to be prepared in wax with full-arch coverage of either upper or lower teeth. A lower appliance must incorporate guiding inclines for upper posterior teeth to

---

*Condylator Service, CH-8028, Zurich, Switzerland.
†Denar Corp., Anaheim, Calif. 92805, USA.

Figure 4.4 Unloading appliance – articulator adjustment.

(a) and (b) Condylar spheres located in the articulator fossa boxes for RP mounting.

(c) and (d) Articulated casts at RP mounting. Pencil line marks mesiobuccal cusp tip of 1.6 and 2.6, and corresponding areas of opposing teeth 4.6 and 3.6 respectively. Teeth 1.6, 4.6 have a second line to mark buccal groove of 1.6 and the corresponding area of 4.6.

(e) and (f) Adjustment of condylar elements of articulator to advance the condylar sphere using the 'centric screw'; and to distract the condylar sphere by placing a 1 mm thick insert against the superior wall of the fossa box bilaterally. Degree of adjustment based on assessment of standardized transcranial radiographs depicting condylar orientation.

(g) and (h) Adjustment of the articulator ((e) and (f)) results in a re-alignment of the articulated study casts. Note the alteration in relative positions of pencil lines

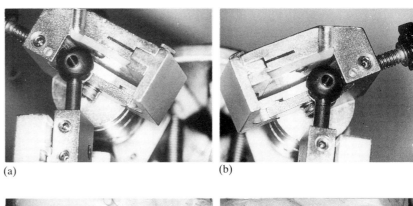

(a)   (b)

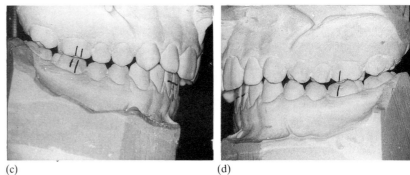

(c)   (d)

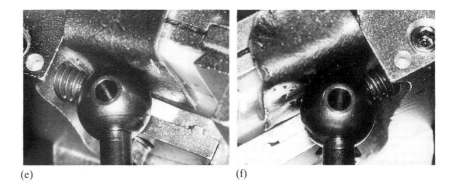

(e)   (f)

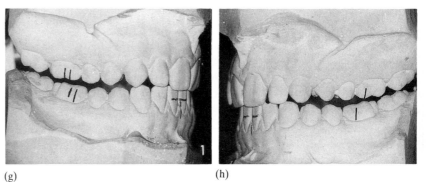

(g)   (h)

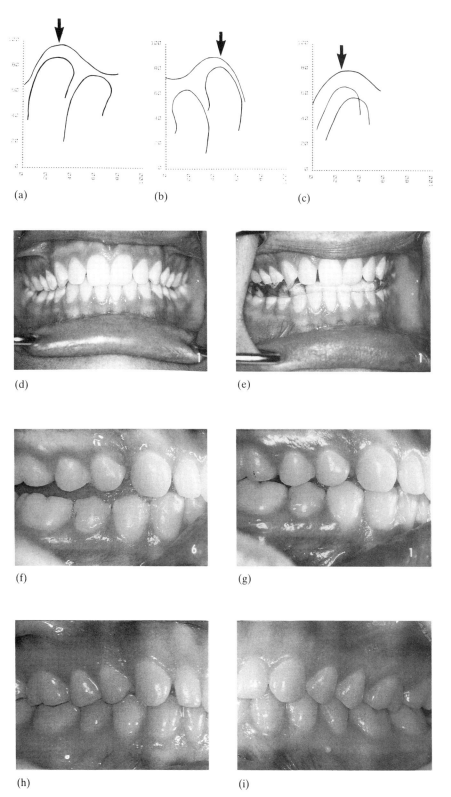

Figure 4.5 Unloading appliance.

(a) and (b) Computer tracings from standardized transcranial radiographs of the TM joint ((a) = Rt and (b) = Lt) showing bilateral change in condyle position from IP (arrow) to a jaw opening of 20 mm (the more anterior tracing).

(c) Computer tracings from standardized transcranial radiographs of the right TM joint showing a change in condyle position from IP (the more posterior position, see arrow) to a more anterior and inferior condyle position following the fitting of an unloading appliance. See text for details.

(d) Intra-oral view of tooth contacts in IP in a patient (SH: ♀, 14 years) with unilateral closed-lock of the right TM joint.

(e) Intra-oral view of the fitted unloading appliance. In this case a mandibular appliance was designed incorporating posterior tooth guide planes to maintain the desired jaw position. The distraction of the right condyle allowed a repositioning of the interarticular disc, and a resolution of symptoms.

(f) Intra-oral view of posterior open bite following the use of an unloading appliance for six weeks (GW: ♀, 15 years) with unilateral closed-lock and pain.

(g) Intra-oral view of posterior teeth of patient shown in (f) showing restoration of molar-bicuspid contacts in IP, following progressive modification of the appliance over a further six weeks. Conservative treatment only is indicated in such cases.

(h) and (i) Intra-oral view of posterior teeth on right and left of patient shown in (f) and (g), six years after completion of treatment. The posterior teeth are now in optimum alignment for function and jaw support. There have been no further episodes of TM joint pain, closed-lock or other dysfunctions.

The use of an unloading appliance allowed physiological re-alignment of interarticular disc and condyle. Progressive adjustment of the appliance allowed gradual eruption of posterior teeth with re-alignment of the TM joints to overcome the posterior open bite that developed as a result of joint unloading. No occlusal adjustment was required

Figure 4.6 Repositioning appliance – technical.

(a) Study casts articulated in RP with an RP transfer record. Note posterior displacement from IP of lower jaw as indicated by position of teeth 1.6 and 4.6; displacement is of the order of 1.0 mm. Compare with (b) and (c).

(b) Study casts articulated in IP. Note position of first molar teeth as indicated by marks drawn on teeth 1.6 and 4.6.

(c) Study casts articulated in a protrusive position with a protrusive transfer record. The anterior jaw position was determined clinically as the first position at which clicking did not occur with jaw opening. Note anterior position of lower jaw as indicated by position of teeth 1.6 and 4.6. In this patient the anterior position of the jaw is of the order of 1.5 mm anterior to IP and 2.5 mm anterior to RP.

(d) Repositioning appliance prepared in wax on the upper teeth following the jaw position described in (c).

(e) Repositioning appliance prepared in wax on the upper teeth. Note lingual 'skirt' extension as the guide plane to maintain the protruded jaw position.

(f) Repositioning appliance prepared in wax on the upper teeth. Note contour of lingual 'skirt' extension that is designed to follow the lingual inclines of the lower teeth. The mandibular cusp tips contact the flat-plane of the splint wax-up; contact points of cusp tips may be seen (arrows)

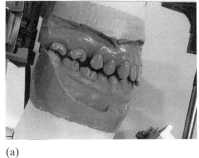

(a)

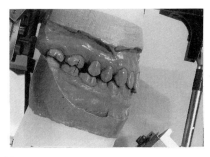

(b)

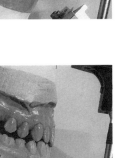

(c)

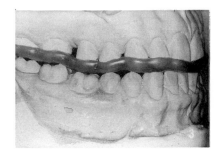

(d)

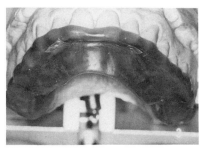

(e)

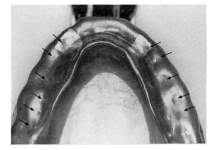

(f)

maintain the appropriate re-alignment of the jaw (Figure 4.5). However, an upper appliance may be made with flat-plane contact against lower teeth and incorporating a lingual 'skirt' extension to maintain lower jaw position (Figure 4.6). This type of appliance is easier to adjust and generally preferred by the author. The wax-up may be refined as required before processing in heat cured acrylic resin.

Such unloading appliances are indicated in a number of acute inflammatory conditions such as the acute phase of degenerative arthrosis (i.e. degenerative arthritis), ankylosing spondylitis, and acute exacerbations of rheumatoid arthritis affecting the TM joints. An unloading appliance may also be indicated where the interarticular disc is displaced anteromedially as 'closed lock' and cannot be re-aligned (or 'recaptured' by jaw manipulation) to restore jaw mobility.

The unloading appliance must be worn full-time during the day, including mealtimes, as well as at night, in order to be effective in helping to resolve the acute intra-articular inflammation and to assist interarticular disc displacement problems. Patient compliance is an important aspect of the success of this treatment.

Following resolution of the acute arthritic episode, a standard flat plane splint may then be used at night only. With disc re-alignment, once the clinical condition of closed-lock has eased and jaw joint mobility has improved, the case must be re-assessed to determine appropriate further treatment. This may require a permanent build up of posterior teeth to maintain jaw re-alignment in the form of a removable overdenture, or re-alignment of posterior teeth orthodontically or with onlays or full crowns.

4.7.2 Repositioning appliances (Figures 4.6, 4.7, 4.8)

This appliance is indicated for treatment of reciprocal TM joint clicking, and is best designed on casts articulated with an anterior or protruded maxillomandibular record. The degree of anterior (or protrusive) jaw re-alignment is determined clinically by instructing the patient to open or protrude the jaw. In so doing, the affected joint (or joints) will click (often causing pain), indicating clinically that the interarticular disc has now become more correctly aligned, with the central bearing surface interposed between the head of the condyle and articular tubercle. It should be emphasized that this is a clinical assessment only, and in order to be more certain of the alignment of interarticular disc and condyle, arthrographic examination of the TM joints is needed, together with fluoroscopy, to be able to examine the dynamics of disc and condyle with jaw movement.

With video recording, it is possible to study the replay and carefully assess disc and condyle function. Following video assessment, it will be clear whether the interarticular disc is fully or partially recaptured at the clinically determined protruded jaw position.

In the absence of this facility, the determination is made clinically:

The patient is instructed to close the jaw slowly and carefully from an opened position or to retrude the jaw from a protruded position, and to

Figure 4.7 Repositioning appliance – clinical.

(a) The extent of jaw opening (interincisor separation of 10 mm) in a patient with closed-lock and unilateral pain of the TM joint.

(b) Maxillary repositioning appliance in place following the preparation described in Figure 4.6.

(c) Maxillary repositioning appliance now allows jaw opening to occur beyond the closed-lock position (compare with (a)).

(d) Following the fitting of a maxillary repositioning appliance, jaw opening of the order of 40 mm inter-incisor separation is now possible, and without pain.

(e) During jaw closing, the lingual skirt extension provides guidance for lower teeth in order to maintain the anterior jaw position.

(f) Maxillary repositioning appliance showing stops for mandibular cusp tips against the flat plane of the occlusal surface. Note guide marks on lingual extension produced during jaw closure

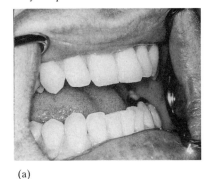

(a)

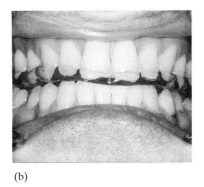

(b)

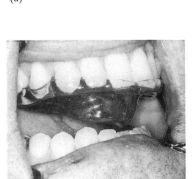

(c)

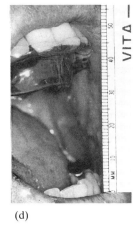

(d)

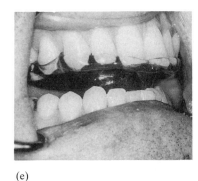

(e)

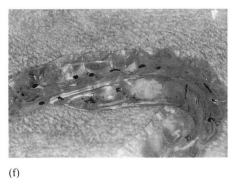

(f)

stop at a point immediately before the click occurs. It is presumed that when the jaw is opened or protruded, the click is associated with the interarticular disc becoming correctly re-aligned (or 'captured'), the click being due to the posterior thick band of the disc passing rapidly over the head of the condyle with protrusion or opening.

Having allowed the disc to re-align itself, the condition is tested by repeating the jaw opening from the protruded position, and this should not evoke either pain or joint sounds.

It is then necessary to capture this protruded jaw position in order to construct an appropriate appliance. An incisal stop may be made in greenstick compound, Optosil* putty or Duralay† to fix the anterior jaw position, and an interocclusal record may then be taken with the anterior stop in place as a guide to jaw position. The casts are articulated with a standard facebow record and a protruded jaw recording. An upper appliance is prepared in baseplate wax with a lingual extension and flat-plane contact against lower teeth to maintain the forward jaw position, allowing jaw opening to occur without clicking. Processing in the customary way is then carried out. Clark (1986) has described the laboratory phases of preparation of repositioning appliances using articulated study casts, and the clinical adjustments required.

It may be more acceptable to the patient, and to ensure that an appliance is worn continuously, for a lower appliance to be used during the day and an upper appliance to be used at night. The lower appliance incorporates indentations of the upper posterior teeth (Figure 4.8) to stabilize the correctly protruded jaw position; the neuromuscular system rapidly adapts to the new intercuspal position.

The appliance is fitted so that it is comfortable; it must be worn continuously during day and night. Once symptoms of clicking, closed-lock or painful crepitus have resolved, usually after four to six weeks, the guiding incline of the lingual extension may be removed progressively to allow a return to the original intercuspal position of the jaw and teeth. The removal of the lingual extension results in the development of the standard splint form.

In *young patients* where symptoms of clicking and particularly reciprocal clicking and/or closed-lock have resolved, this type of appliance therapy may then be reinforced by isokinetic exercises (see Chapter 2 for patient instruction information and Figure 2.1), in order to retrain jaw muscle coordination once the re-alignment of the interarticular disc has been achieved. In young patients, the treatment plan is to return the jaw to its original position with posterior tooth contact over a two to three month period. This may be achieved by progressive reduction of the guide plane or inclines which slowly allows the jaw to retrude without the click recurring. This re-aligning allows the compressed posterior attachment tissues in young individuals to repair, so that optimal function of articular tissues can be re-established with a return to the original intercuspal jaw position.

In young patients requiring orthodontic treatment, a combination of orthodontic and orthopaedic treatment may allow optimum posterior tooth alignment with anterior jaw repositioning (Festa, 1985; Owen, 1984a,b, 1985). This has been shown to encourage condylar growth and remodelling to develop a stable condyle–interarticular disc relationship in a variety of clinical conditions (Festa, 1985; Mongini and Schmid, 1987).

In *older patients* where symptoms of crepitus and/or closed-lock are present in conjunction with degenerative changes in articular tissues,

*Bayer AG, D5090 Leverkusen, Germany.
†Reliance Dental Mfg Co., Worth, Ill. 60482, USA.

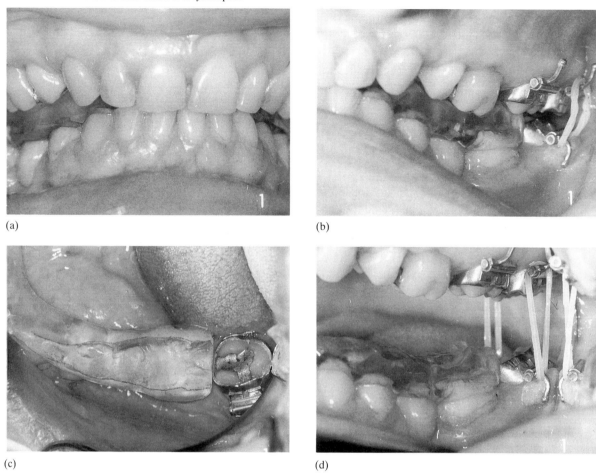

(a)

(b)

(c)

(d)

Figure 4.8

(a) Intra-oral view of lower repositioning appliance in position to re-align the jaw and manage the internal joint derangement. Indications: reciprocal clicking, pain, limited jaw opening, and deviation to ipsilateral side where symptoms were acute. Patient ♀, 36 years was maintained pain-free with repositioning appliance for 12 months.

(b) Definitive treatment in progress following pain relief and management of internal derangement: Orthodontic treatment to extrude posterior teeth progressively. In this illustration, second molar teeth and upper first molar have orthodontic bands and elastic traction on second molars to

secondary treatment should be delayed for at least two or three months following primary treatment for pain dysfunction. If it is not possible to regain the original jaw position and posterior tooth contacts by progressive reduction of the guide planes on the appliance, it will be necessary to stabilize the posterior jaw support in some way. This may involve fixed or removable restorations or orthodontic re-alignment of posterior teeth to permanently maintain jaw support at the re-aligned jaw position. This has now become an attractive treatment alternative for appropriate adult patients (Miller, 1988).

Summary

There is a regular need for occlusal splints in prosthodontic treatment planning and in the management of craniomandibular dysfunction and pain. In order for such appliances to be effective, they must be designed correctly and regularly adjusted following initial fitting. In the management of pain dysfunctions, additional treatment is often required following resolution of symptoms to stabilize jaw position and to remove posterior tooth contact interferences if present. The latter may result in torque forces developing around such interferences during the tooth contact phase of jaw function and/or parafunction, which may lead to the development of muscle pain. Long-term follow-up is essential, however, before any claims may be made concerning the effectiveness of this type of therapy.

Whether occlusal splints have a potentiating effect on general muscle performance in sport requires further investigation; however, it appears that there may be some sports (weight lifting) where this may be so. There is no doubt, however, that occlusal splints, if correctly designed and maintained, have a generally beneficial effect on muscle function.

There are limits to the use of the standard splint in management of the occlusion, and for particular clinical dysfunctions an anterior repositioning or an unloading appliance may be indicated.

4.8 Use and care of occlusal splints

The following information is written as a hand-out for patients. It is important for them to be able to refer to these details during the early period of splint use when they may be uncertain of their maintenance responsibilities. As well, it emphasizes the need for splint adjustment and the importance of supervision by a dentist.

INFORMATION FOR PATIENTS
USE AND CARE OF OCCLUSAL SPLINTS

Your occlusal splint is designed to relieve muscle tension, decrease painful symptoms, protect the teeth, and maintain the teeth in position. The following information will help you in using the splint correctly:

The splint should be worn as much as possible, except when eating.

At first you may be aware of an increase in the amount of saliva in your mouth. This is normal and will disappear after several days.

When placed in your mouth, the splint may feel tight on your teeth for a short time.

When the splint is removed, your teeth may feel different, and when the teeth are brought together the interferences that are present may temporarily seem greater. This is common and will disappear.

The splint must be stored in water to preserve the plastic. When carrying the splint, keep it wrapped in moist tissue in a plastic container.

The splint should be brushed with a tooth brush and toothpaste after meals and before bed.

Adjustments of the splint are always necessary and the number needed will depend on the nature, complexity, and severity of your joint-muscle problem.

If the splint is not used, symptoms may return or become worse.

In addition to splint therapy, an occlusal adjustment of your teeth may be necessary to provide more effective therapy. This will be decided after the splint has eliminated the symptoms.

Figure 4.8 (*cont.*)
extrude these teeth. The appliance has been reduced to allow second molar movement whilst maintaining treatment jaw position.

(c) Lower appliance in place with reduced posterior extension to allow second molar movement. Note contour of lower appliance to allow full time use – narrow occlusal table with minimal extension bucco-lingually.

(d) Elastic traction designed to extrude second molar teeth.

This dysfunction was one of chronic internal derangement. Clinical assessment and management with repositioning appliance over 12 months confirmed that permanent stabilization was desirable in this case (see Chapter 2.5 for further details)

The splint should not be worn unless you are under the supervision of a dentist. If you move from your present home or discontinue treatment, *do not* continue to wear the splint without consulting a dentist.

References

Ash, M. M. and Ramfjord, S. P. (1982) *An Introduction to Functional Occlusion*, W. B. Saunders, Philadelphia, pp. 181–207

Clark, G. T. (1986) The TMJ repositioning appliance: a technique for construction, insertion and adjustment. *Journal of Craniomandibular Practice*, **4**, 37–46

Eversaul, G. A. (1977) Applied kinesiology and the treatment of TMJ dysfunction. In *Clinical Management of Head, Neck and TMJ Pain and Dysfunction* (ed. H. Gelb), W. B. Saunders, Philadelphia, pp. 480–506

Farrar, W. B. (1972) Differentiation of temporomandibular joint dysfunction to simplify treatment. *Journal of Prosthetic Dentistry*, **28**, 629–635

Festa, F. (1985) Joint distraction and condyle advancement with a modified functional distraction appliance. *Journal of Craniomandibular Practice*, **3**, 344–350

Gelb, H. (1977) Effective management and treatment of the craniomandibular syndrome. In *Clinical Management of Head, Neck and TMJ Pain and Dysfunction* (ed. H. Gelb), W. B. Saunders, Philadelphia, pp. 288–369

Gibbs, C. H., Messerman, T., Reswick, J. B. and Derda, H. J. (1971) Functional movements of the mandible. *Journal of Prosthetic Dentistry*, **26**, 604–620

Gibbs, C. H., Lundeen, A. C., Mahan, P. E. and Fujimoto, J. (1981) Chewing movements in relation to border movements at the first molar. *Journal of Prosthetic Dentistry*, **46**, 308–322

Goldspink, G. (1976) The adaptation of muscle to a new functional length. In *Mastication* (eds D. J. Anderson and B. Matthews), John Wright, Bristol, pp. 90–99

Greenberg, M. S., Cohen, S. G., Springer, P. *et al.* (1981) Mandibular position and upper body strength: a controlled clinical trial. *Journal of the American Dental Association*, **103**, 576–579

Hawley, C. A. (1919) Removable retainer. *International Journal of Orthodontia*, **5**, 291–305

Heir, G. M., Berrett, A. and Worth, D. A. (1983) Diagnosis and management of TMJ involvement in ankylosing spondylitis. *Journal of Craniomandibular Practice*, **1**, 75–81

Ingervall, B. and Carlsson, G. E. (1982) Masticatory muscle activity before and after elimination of balancing side occlusal interferences. *Journal of Oral Rehabilitation*, **9**, 183–192

Ingervall, B. and Thilander, B. (1974) Relation between facial morphology and activity of the masticatory muscles. *Journal of Oral Rehabilitation*, **1**, 131–147

Jakush, J. (1982) Can dental therapy enhance athletic performance? *Journal of the American Dental Association*, **104**, 292–298

Klineberg, I. (1980) Influences of temporomandibular articular mechanoreceptors on functional jaw movements. *Journal of Oral Rehabilitation*, **7**, 307–317

Klineberg, I. (1983) Occlusal splints: a critical assessment of their use in prosthodontics. *Australian Dental Journal*, **28**, 1–8

Krogh-Poulsen, W. G. (1969) Management of the occlusion of the teeth. II Examination, diagnosis and treatment. In *Facial Pain and Mandibular Dysfunction* (eds L. Schwartz and C. M. Chayes), W. B. Saunders, Philadelphia, pp. 271–277

Lous, I., Sheikholeslam, A. and Møller, E. (1970) Postural activity in subjects with functional disorders of the chewing apparatus. *Scandinavian Journal of Dental Research*, **78**, 404–410

McNamara, D. C. (1976) Inhibitory effects in masticatory neuromusculature of human subjects at median occlusal position. *Archives of Oral Biology*, **21**, 329–331

McNamara, D. C. (1978) The clinical significance of medial occlusal position. *Journal of Oral Rehabilitation*, **5**, 173–186

Miller, T. E. (1988) Adult orthodontics as an adjunct to restorative care. *International Journal of Prosthodontics*, **1**, 165–174

Møller, E. (1966) The chewing apparatus. *Acta Physiologica Scandinavica*, **69** (Suppl. 280)

Mongini, F. and Schmid, W. (1987) Treatment of mandibular asymmetries during growth. A longitudinal study. *European Journal of Orthodontics,* **9**, 51–67

Nordström, S. H. and Yemm, R. (1972) Sarcomere length in the masseter muscle of the rat. *Archives of Oral Biology,* **17**, 895–902

Nordström, S. H. and Yemm, R. (1974) The relationship between jaw position and isometric active tension produced by direct stimulation of the rat masseter muscle. *Archives of Oral Biology,* **19**, 353–359

Owen, A. H. (1984a) Orthodontic/orthopaedic treatment of craniomandibular pain dysfunction. Part 1: Diagnosis with transcranial radiographs. *Journal of Craniomandibular Practice,* **2**, 239–249

Owen, A. H. (1984b) Orthodontic/orthopaedic treatment of craniomandibular pain dysfunction. Part 2: Posterior condylar displacement. *Journal of Craniomandibular Practice,* **2**, 333–349

Owen, A. H. (1985) Orthodontic/orthopaedic treatment of craniomandibular pain dysfunction. Part 3: Anterior condylar displacement. *Journal of Craniomandibular Practice,* **3**, 31–45

Palla, S. (1979) Diagnosis and therapy of TMJ pain and muscle dysfunction. In *Proceedings of the Second International Prosthodontic Congress* (ed. W. Lefkowitz), C. V. Mosby, St Louis, pp. 282–284

Ringqvist, M. (1973) Isometric bite force and its relation to dimensions of the facial skeleton. *Acta Odontologica Scandinavica,* **31**, 35–42

Thexton, A. J. and Hiiemae, K. (1975) The twitch tension characteristics of opossum jaw musculature. *Archives of Oral Biology,* **20**, 743–748

Timm, T. A. and Ash, M. M. (1977) The occlusal bite plane splint: an adjunct to orthodontic treatment. *Journal of Clinical Orthodontics,* **11**, 383–390

Troelstrup, B. and Møller, E. (1970) Electromyography of the temporalis and masseter muscles in children with unilateral cross-bite. *Scandinavian Journal of Dental Research,* **78**, 425–430

Wallace, C. J. and Klineberg, I. (1990) Splint therapy for craniocervical dysfunction. *Journal of Dental Research,* **69** (Abstr. 21): 935

Wilkes, C. H. (1978) Structural and functional alterations of the temporomandibular joint. *North-west Dentistry,* **57**, 287–294

Yemm, R. (1979) Neurophysiologic studies of temporomandibular joint dysfunction. In *Temporomandibular Joint Function and Dysfunction* (eds G. A. Zarb and G. E. Carlsson), Munksgaard, Copenhagen, pp. 215–237

Chapter 5

Occlusal adjustment procedures

5.1 Introduction

Occlusal adjustment is a procedure where selective areas of tooth cusp inclines, marginal ridges and transverse ridges are modified to provide improved tooth and jaw stability and to direct loading onto appropriate teeth during lateral excursions. This procedure should be a routine requirement in general restorative treatment and particularly where complex prosthodontic procedures are to be undertaken. Occlusal adjustment procedures should be regarded as preventive therapy for the occlusion, to promote harmonious function of jaw muscles, TM joints and teeth, in a way similar to that in which plaque control and toothbrush instruction is a routine preventive measure essential to gingival health. Improved neuromuscular harmony following occlusal adjustment procedures has been described (McNamara, 1976, 1977). Although mock adjustment (Goodman, Greene and Laskin, 1976; Forssell, Kirveskari and Kangasniemi, 1986, 1987) and occlusal adjustment were found to be equally effective in relieving symptoms of dysfunction, there was a significantly greater reduction in clinical signs of dysfunction where true adjustment was carried out.

Table 5.1 summarizes the general goals desirable for management of the occlusion independent of the procedure to be undertaken. Thus, irrespective of whether the treatment to follow involves fitting an occlusal splint, carrying out an occlusal adjustment, or restoring teeth with simple restorations or complex reconstructions, the fundamental criteria to be satisfied should be the same.

The dynamic interplay of teeth, TM joints and jaw muscles is complex. However, the teeth play a critical role in influencing the way jaw muscles function, so that in order to maintain long-term stability of the system, it is necessary for intra- and interarch tooth relationships to promote smooth synchronous muscle activity and jaw translation. Satisfying the requirements of Table 5.1 will allow this to be achieved in restorative treatment.

Table 5.1 Management of the occlusion – general philosophy

INTRA-ARCH STABILITY:
  Flat occlusal plane anteroposteriorly, minimum lateral curve

INTER-ARCH STABILITY:
  Bilateral synchronous contacts on posterior teeth in IP and RP, at the correct vertical dimension of occlusion;
  Guidance for lateral and protrusive jaw movements on anterior teeth, or as far anteriorly as possible to provide anterior 'freedom' for functional jaw movements close to IP. Where possible, the canine teeth should provide this guidance and allow easy gliding movements in forward and lateral directions

OPTIMUM ANTERIOR TOOTH ARRANGEMENT:
  Lip support for aesthetics and speech;
  Tongue function for speech and mastication.
  Acceptable overbite and overjet (for anterior guidance)

TM JOINT:
  Optimum disc: condyle relationship for fluent joint translation and rotation

5.2 General considerations

5.2.1 Reversible or irreversible therapy

Occlusal therapies may be either reversible or irreversible.

Reversible procedures include occlusal stabilization splints and physical therapies such as jaw exercises, jaw manipulation and other physiotherapy treatments.

Irreversible therapies include a variety of treatments such as occlusal repositioning appliances, orthodontic treatment, orthognathic surgery, fixed and removable prosthodontic treatment and occlusal adjustment. Because of the irreversible nature of these procedures, there must be precise indications of the advantages of such changes. It is clear that where there are jaw and alveolar bone discrepancies resulting in functional and aesthetic problems, the indications for major treatment are obvious to the clinician and often enthusiastically requested by the patient.

In this way, the outcome of orthognathic surgery and orthodontic treatment is usually predictable and successful if clinically justified for aesthetic or functional reasons. Similarly, the indications for fixed and removable prosthodontic treatment are usually obvious and sought after by the patient.

5.2.2 Indications for occlusal adjustment

In the case of occlusal adjustment, the indications must be apparent to the operator and the benefits clearly understood by the patient. The clinician must explain precisely what is meant by the procedure, how the procedure is to be carried out in each stage and the advantages to the patient. The use of articulated study casts allows the reasons for the procedure and the advantages to be clearly described to the patient.

Indications for occlusal adjustment include:

1. Pre-treatment in prosthodontic and general restorative care:
   - to improve jaw relationships and provide stable tooth contacts for jaw support in IP; and
   - to improve the stability of individual teeth.
2. Enhancement of function by providing smooth directional guidance for lateral and protrusive jaw movements. This may involve the modification of plunger cusps, inlocking cuspal inclines, non-working supracontacts and the like.
3. Traumatic occlusion where supracontacts associated with excessive tooth loading, such as may occur in parafunctional clenching, result in tooth sensitivity and increased tooth mobility.
4. Stabilizing or correcting previous orthodontic, restorative or prosthodontic treatment. In such cases where it is decided that the restorations are to be retained, an occlusal adjustment may be indicated. Alternatively, adjustment in conjunction with occlusal build-up on selected teeth may be required.

5.2.3 The special nature of orofacial pain

Where occlusal adjustment is to be carried out as a treatment for orofacial pain and neuromuscular dysfunction of jaw muscles and TM joints, the situation is quite different. Under these circumstances occlusal splint therapy is an essential pre-treatment diagnostic aid. This is especially so in the case of chronic orofacial pain problems (the problem is regarded as 'chronic' if it has been present without relief for some months – Sternbach, 1974), where the psychopathology has become altered by the duration of suffering. In acute orofacial pain dysfunction (present for hours or days), the problem of the patient's altered psychopathology usually does not arise, and there may be obvious indications for occlusal adjustment.

However, in most instances there are other aetiological factors superimposed on the dental condition (occlusal irregularities associated with centric and eccentric tooth relationships). In most cases the dental status has existed unchanged for some time before the onset of pain or dysfunction.

Occlusal irregularities, particularly tooth contact interferences between IP(CO) and RP(CR), mediotrusive (non-working) interferences and protrusive interferences are usually considered by dentists to be of aetiological importance in parafunction (tooth clenching or grinding) and orofacial pain and dysfunction. These conclusions are based on empirical evidence only, and there is no documented scientific evidence from controlled clinical trials (Matthews, 1975; Yemm, 1979; Barghi, Rugh and Drago, 1979; Bailey and Rugh, 1980), to directly link occlusal irregularities with the aetiology of parafunction. There is some evidence however that occlusal irregularities may be related to jaw muscle pain and TM joint dysfunction (for further details see Chapter 2, Section 2.4), by their effects on directional guidance of the teeth in function. Also, mock occlusal adjustment has been shown to be effective in reducing pain dysfunction (Goodman, Greene and Laskin, 1976). Clark and Adler (1985) reviewed the efficacy of occlusal adjustment procedures and concluded that no comparative studies have indicated that any one of the commonly used techniques is superior to another, that occlusal interferences may affect periodontal tissues, and that dental treatment which interferes with intercuspal contact also alters postural muscle activity and may thus cause pain and dysfunction.

5.2.4 Psychopathological considerations

It is important to acknowledge that because of the psychosocial significance of orofacial structures in growth and development, occlusal adjustment is a psychophysical therapy. As a result of the uncertain outcome of occlusal adjustment in some patients, it is not indicated in the primary management of orofacial pain. This problem arises because of the variability in stereognostic sense (or discriminative ability to detect small changes in tooth contacts). The discriminative sense varies in some individuals from being able to detect foil as fine as 5μ placed between contacting teeth to not being able to detect foil of 80μ thickness or more between the teeth in other individuals.

The significance of this discriminative sense is that the patient with an acute discriminative sense may never be 'comfortable' in IP (centric) after occlusal adjustment (see Chapter 2, Section 2.2.3(d)).

Stereognostic sense arises from the especially rich sensory and motor innervation of orofacial structures and the unique psychosocial and psychosexual importance of the face and mouth to the individual. As a result of this complex psychophysiological interplay, it is difficult for the patient to correctly judge the degree of alteration made to teeth (i.e. the amount of tooth structure removed in an adjustment), and all patients tend to magnify the effects (i.e. they imagine a greater amount of tooth structure has been removed). In extreme cases a delusional state may result.

The psychiatric conditions of 'monosymptomatic hypochondriacal psychosis', indicating a distorted body image, or 'dysmorphophobia', which includes the complaint of a cosmetic defect (where the patient is convinced that the change has altered their appearance), are known to be associated with alterations to the teeth (see Chapter 2, Section 2.2.3(e) for further information). This problem may also be due to the fact that the patient is unable to see the alterations to the teeth following an occlusal adjustment. In other more severe forms of irreversible occlusal therapy, particularly crown and bridge work, the alterations are usually clearly visible to the patient, and this is reassuring if the work is completed to a high standard. However, in the latter cases, those patients with an acute stereognostic sense may complain that their 'bite' has been altered, particularly if the treatment has caused changes to IP and been carried out to a poor standard, and such patients may also develop a delusional psychotic disorder. This situation becomes untreatable, and motivates such patients to continue to seek dental help in order to restore their 'bite'. This morbid preoccupation with the teeth and the alterations made to them is termed 'phantom bite' (Marbach, 1976, 1978; Munro, 1978; Marbach *et al.*, 1983). The patient with a less acute stereognostic sense may not detect fine irregularities or changes in tooth contact and generally would not be as critical of dental treatment carried out.

The indication for occlusal adjustment must thus follow the successful use of an occlusal splint as primary treatment in relieving symptoms. Following splint therapy, many patients will describe a difference in the quality of tooth contacts (the 'bite') with the splint in place and immediately after the splint is removed. This difference is due to the altered jaw position induced by the splint with jaw muscles reprogrammed to accommodate a new functional tooth contact position (i.e. against the splint surface). This new tooth contact pattern may be adjusted following assessment of articulated study casts, but the difference in the 'bite' does not necessarily indicate cause and effect in relation to a presenting pain problem.

5.3 Occlusal adjustment philosophies

A number of approaches to occlusal adjustment have been proposed on the basis of:

1. The position of the mandible at which the occlusal adjustment is carried out;
2. Lateral and protrusive guidance; and
3. The occlusal contact scheme.

5.3.1 Mandibular position

1. The retruded jaw position or centric relation jaw position has been presented as the optimum functional jaw position where RP is coincident with IP. This was part of a philosophy developed by B. B. McCollum (1955), who was the prime mover and leading figure in the development of a new and comprehensive approach to clinical treatment which was termed 'gnathology'. The genesis of this new development centred around the Study Club of California and included prominent clinicians of the time, amongst them Charles Stuart, Harvey Stallard and Peter K. Thomas.

   These clinicians actively promoted the gnathology philosophy and this has had a profound influence on dental treatment and especially fixed prosthodontic treatment in North America. In addition and as an integral part of the philosophy, the need was perceived for the development of fully adjustable instrumentation including articulators and pantographs. The Stuart* fully adjustable articulator and pantograph have since been regarded as essential for clinical accuracy by followers of the gnathology philosophy.

   This development may be applauded as possibly the most significant attempt to understand the management of the jaw muscle system. However, in more recent times, clinicians have become preoccupied with instrumentation. The development of a far too mechanistic approach to the management of a biological system has unfortunately undermined the real significance of the original gnathology philosophy. Also, commercial interests in the development and promotion of articulators and pantographs have presented a biased view, further alienating many academics and clinicians who appreciate the essential need for understanding the biology of the occlusal system. The system should be seen to be complex, variable and adaptable and limited by anatomical and physiological constraints.
2. The retruded jaw position or centric relation jaw position is a reference position for transfer records and there should be freedom for tooth contacts forward of RP. This 'long centric' philosophy has been described and promoted by Pankey (see Mann and Pankey, 1963) and Dawson (1989).
3. Retruded jaw position or centric relation jaw position is a reference position for transfer records and IP is the functional tooth position with

---

*C. E. Stuart Gnathological Instruments, Ventura, Calif. 93001, USA.

freedom for lateral, protrusive and retrusive jaw movements from IP. This 'freedom in centric' philosophy has been described and promoted as more physiological by Schuyler (1935), Beyron (1954) and Ramfjord and Ash (1983).

5.3.2 Excursive guidance

1. Balanced occlusion – this is desirable in complete denture construction to help stabilize the lower denture, particularly during function once the food bolus has been penetrated. It is also indicated in severely compromised dentitions with marked tooth mobility.
2. Canine guidance is considered an essential requirement by the 'gnathology' group and the 'freedom in centric' group.
3. Group function is considered an optimum requirement in the 'long centric' philosophy.

   Ingervall and Hedegård (1974) found that, in 85% of natural dentitions, there were balancing contacts and interferences; guidance on canines was found to occur in 40%, on bicuspids in 20% and on molars in 10% of cases. This does not imply, however, that in occlusal therapy these features should be reproduced, and clinical experience has suggested that in reconstructed cases the occlusal scheme should be different.

   Clinical experience indicates the desirability of developing anterior guidance involving canine, or canine and bicuspid teeth. This clinical assessment has been shown to be advantageous in a series of physiological studies (Bakke, Møller and Thorsen, 1980, 1982; MacDonald and Hannam, 1984; Manns, Chan and Miralles, 1987).

5.3.3 Occlusal contact scheme

1. Tripodized cusp support – 'point' centric philosophy, as described by McCollum (1955) and Stuart (see Stuart and Stallard, 1960).
2. Cusp-fossa, cusp-marginal ridge – 'freedom' in centric philosophy, as described by Schuyler (1935), Beyron (1954) and Ramfjord and Ash (1983).
3. Cusp-fossa, marginal ridge – 'long' centric philosophy, as described by Mann and Pankey (1963) and Dawson (1989).

   It would appear from an assessment of the various philosophies and tooth contact characteristics that, once condyle position is determined, and once lateral and protrusive guidance is determined, the contact scheme of bicuspid and molar teeth is of secondary importance. It is the author's opinion that the preoccupations of some occlusal philosophies with tripodized cusp contact form is unnecessary from the viewpoints of jaw support, functional harmony of muscles–joints–teeth and functional efficiency.

5.4 Goals of occlusal adjustment

These goals may be achieved by developing a cusp-fossa, and/or cusp-marginal ridge tooth contact arrangement. Also, 'freedom' for smooth anteroposterior and lateral jaw movement is necessary between IP and the guiding influence of the anterior teeth.

Anterior guidance is an important component of a harmonious neuromuscular system; however, the nature of the guidance is important. The presence of 'anterior interference' is not uncommon, where the anterior guidance is not in harmony with function and anterior tooth mobility may be detected clinically. This must be carefully checked in clinical assessment by observing and palpating upper anterior teeth with jaw clenching. Mobility without bone loss indicates interference. This is often present with a 'deep' or a 'closed' bite anteriorly in the absence of anterior 'freedom' in jaw movement.

In general, goals in the short term are to eliminate gross occlusal interferences that develop:

1. Along the arc of jaw closure associated with plunger cusps from extruded, drifted and tilted teeth. This is especially important where there is a distal jaw displacement and/or a wedging effect locking the jaw in centric; and
2. Lateral interferences on posterior teeth that develop as working or non-working interferences associated with a steep lateral curve (curve of Wilson). This may result from extrusion and rotation of posterior teeth from undercontoured restorations, absence of adequate opposing teeth, and parafunctional wear.

In the long term the goals are to establish and maintain a healthy, comfortable, functioning, stable dentition.

In the intact dentition it will be possible to provide a refined occlusal contact scheme by satisfying the criteria detailed below. However, once teeth are lost, the partially dentate situation is more complex to manage and may require gross adjustment in conjunction with the addition of tooth material (adhesive restorations or, where indicated, onlays or crowns) in conjunction with removable prostheses.

Goals may be listed as follows:

1. To provide simultaneous bilateral contacts on two or more posterior teeth in RP and in MOP.
2. To provide freedom for the jaw to move from RP without posterior interferences or contacts in excursive movements.
3. To increase the functional angle of occlusion (FAO) (Figure 5.1).
4. To aid pre-treatment in restorative dentistry particularly involving removable partial dentures, fixed prosthodontics and fixed-removable restorations.
5. As adjunctive therapy in the treatment of joint-muscle pain dysfunction, where there is occlusal instability (i.e. an absence of bilateral contacts on posterior teeth. This is often brought about by missing teeth with drifting and extrusion of adjacent teeth into the space or a tooth arrangement which restricts the FAO, such as a deep anterior overbite with minimal overjet), which has an aetiological role. Such occlusal problems may lead to:

– intra-articular degenerative changes due to joint loading affecting articular eminence, interarticular disc and condyle;

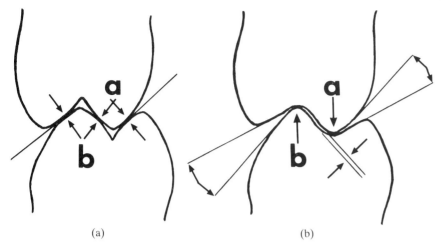

(a)   (b)

Figure 5.1 Diagrammatic representation of a buccolingual view of a cross-section through the mid-cusp area showing supporting cusps (maxillary lingual – **a**; mandibular buccal – **b**) and non-supporting cusps (maxillary buccal, mandibular lingual).

(a) Represents the type of contact which may be seen where multiple contacts between opposing cusps (arrows) occur, dictating one position of intercuspation. The steepness of the cuspal inclines limits the FAO.

(b) Represents cuspal contact following occlusal adjustment where a cusp-fossa relationship is developed for maxillary lingual cusps and opposing fossae, and mandibular buccal cusps and opposing fossae. Also, the steepness of the non-supporting cuspal inclines has been reduced, and, where necessary, the buccal incline of the mandibular supporting cusp. These latter adjustments increase the FAO (as indicated) so that there is a wider approach angle into and away from tooth contact, and there is thus an increased 'freedom' around tooth contact

– phasic changes in evoked jaw muscle reflexes; and
– tonic changes in coordinated jaw muscle activity.

5.5 Significance of a 'slide in centric'

This may be explained by considering the following:
1. It had been proposed, initially by Ramfjord (1961), that the slide from IP to RP was a potential problem as a 'trigger' for bruxism. This was repeated by other authors and accepted in general, although the original evidence was inconclusive, and it is now considered that tooth contact interferences do not trigger bruxism.
2. The slide and its association with the TM joint: Firstly, in correlating form and function, it is clear that the anterior slope of the condyle and posterior slope of the eminence (or articular tubercle) with the disc interposed are the functional joint surfaces. This is particularly obvious from the thickened covering of shear-resistant fibrous tissue present in these areas to cope with joint rotation and translation, as well as the relative bone thickness of fossa and tubercle.

   Secondly, it is also known that during the final closing phase of jaw movement in function, the upper head of the lateral pterygoid muscle is active and helps stabilize disc and condyle in apposition with the posterior slope of the eminence. During this power stroke phase, mesially directed tooth guidance will ensure that this relationship (of condyle disc and eminence) is maintained. This is enhanced by guidance on mesial inclines of posterior teeth initially and then mesially directed anterior tooth guidance. Thus, an anterior 'slide in centric', which directs the jaw forwards and does not have a steep vertical component, encourages apposition of condyle, disc and eminence during the power stroke of jaw closing. The author considers, from clinical experience, that this type of 'slide in centric' should NOT be eliminated, as it appears to have a protective role for the joint. Removal of this guidance may allow the condyle to become more posteriorly aligned and this may lead to an unstable disc–condyle relationship with movement of the disc away from the eminence. This situation may predispose to anterior disc displacement.

The important considerations for retaining the 'slide in centric' are that it is well tolerated by the patient, and that tooth contact occurs bilaterally and directs the jaw forwards without a significant lateral displacement. Clinical studies (Sheikholeslam, Møller and Lous, 1982) have shown that occlusal treatment with resolution of craniomandibular pain results in the development of symmetrical jaw muscle activity. It is clear, however, that a number of other factors may contribute to jaw muscle asymmetry (Lund and Widmer, 1989) including age, sex, facial morphology and bruxism. Sherman (1985) studied patients with CMDs with and without a history of bruxism and found that resting masseter EMG activity was far higher in the presence of bruxism.

More recently, Nielsen *et al.* (1990) have shown that following treatment for jaw muscle pain, lateral and protrusive jaw movements became more symmetrical. This writer considers that in the absence of facial asymmetry, optimum jaw function is associated with reasonably symmetrical jaw movement, whilst in the presence of TM joint dysfunction and jaw muscle pain, asymmetrical lateral, protrusive and opening movements will occur.

5.6 Contraindications

1. The presence of an occlusal scheme where, following attrition and erosion, teeth are locked at IP and where there is a possible loss of vertical dimension of occlusion. In such cases tooth addition rather than reduction is indicated.
2. In a patient who is preoccupied with his/her teeth, mouth, bite (i.e. who has a heightened occlusal sense). This is particularly important where previous dental treatment, such as fixed prosthodontics and/or occlusal adjustment, has been unsuccessful in the patient's view.
3. Where the anatomical jaw relationship requires alternative treatment.

5.7 Preclinical procedures

1. Occlusal adjustment is facilitated by initially carrying out the procedure on study casts articulated on an adjustable articulator. The adjustment of casts should:

(a) Eliminate unilateral interferences in mandibular closure but not eliminate a bilaterally symmetrical contact slide which directs the jaw straight forwards into IP;
(b) Provide smooth gliding lateral and protrusive movements.

2. Adjustment of study casts

(a) There are advantages in making an occlusal adjustment on casts, in that details of cusp contacts and tooth inclination are clear. The adjustment in the mouth may vary slightly, however, because of the limitations of the articulator in precisely duplicating mandibular movements. The detection of mediotrusive or non-working and laterotrusive or working contacts or interferences in the mouth often depends on digital palpation of the contacting teeth to determine heavy contacts and/or tooth movement. A non-working interference causes disclusion of the working side, and may easily be seen on articulated casts.

However, in the mouth, a tooth in non-working interference may move at tooth contact, and as a result disclusion will still occur. Occlusal trauma is a common cause of tooth mobility in the absence of periodontal disease and bone loss. The non-working interference becomes a non-working contact as the tooth moves, and anterior guidance may still be present. This is misleading, since tooth mobility would have arisen initially as a result of the interference. Such a situation would be clearly apparent on articulated casts. Thus the detection of non-working or working interferences in the mouth requires tactile as well as visual assessment.

In a study of tooth mobility associated with non-working side interferences, Moozeh, Suit and Bissada (1981) examined the effects of complete elimination of non-working interferences, compared with adjustment to produce non-working contacts only. Thirty-three healthy adults were involved and divided into three groups of eleven each – one group had non-working interferences completely eliminated; in the second group the non-working interferences were adjusted to be harmonious contacts in lateral excursions; and the third group was the control where there was no occlusal adjustment. It was found that the greatest reduction in tooth mobility occurred with complete elimination of the non-working interferences.

(b) On the working side, the contact of one or two teeth is sometimes considered to be an interference. However, contacts on individual teeth are not interferences unless:

(i)   The involved teeth have increased mobility and/or loss of support;
(ii) It is desired to distribute occlusal forces over more teeth; and
(iii) The tooth contacts interfere with or prevent smooth gliding movements of the mandible.

GROSS REMOVAL OF TOOTH STRUCTURE TO OBTAIN MULTIPLE CONTACTS IS CONTRAINDICATED.

(c) As non-working interferences are reduced, increased contacts may occur on the working side (bicuspid, canine, lateral and/or central incisors). A reduction of the canine to increase posterior contacts can result in excessive contacts on bicuspid and incisor teeth.

A REDUCTION OF CANINE, BICUSPID AND INCISOR TEETH, TO INCREASE POSTERIOR CONTACTS OR PROMOTE GROUP FUNCTION, IS CONTRAINDICATED.

(d) In protrusive movements there should be no posterior tooth contacts other than the mandibular first premolars. In the presence of an anterior open-bite, posterior teeth provide guidance which should be smooth. Although canine guidance is desired, EXCESSIVE TOOTH REDUCTION IS CONTRAINDICATED.

It may be necessary to build up the lingual contour of the canine to provide appropriate guidance and an acceptable FAO. This may be carried out in a diagnostic way with composite resin, as a means of assessing the guidance developed. Subsequently, permanent restoration may be carried out with confidence.

The goal is smooth gliding movements on casts as well as in the mouth. However, in the mouth, palpation of the central incisors will often demonstrate slight movement with protrusive and lateral-protrusive movements. A reduction of this movement is desired, but not through the use of excessive tooth adjustment. Adjustment for anterior protrusive interferences is generally carried out by increasing the lingual concavity on the maxillary anterior teeth. Posterior protrusive contacts should be reduced on cusp ridges and triangular ridges, not on cusp tips.

(e) Retruded jaw position
Location of premature contacts:
When moving the mandible into RP, the horizontal overlap of the maxillary arch over the mandibular arch increases. This is shown in Figures 5.2(a) and 5.3(b).

(i)   Depending on the degree of tooth rotation, if any, and the shape of the arch (ovoid, tapering, square), premature contacts occur most often on the LINGUAL INCLINES OF THE BUCCAL CUSPS OF THE MANDIBULAR TEETH.
These premature contacts involve the distal inclines of the triangular ridges. The more tapering the arch, the greater the distal displacement, and the greater the buccal inclination of the maxillary molars and bicuspids, the contact in RP will be higher toward the cusp tip on the mandibular molar.

(ii) Premature contact in RP commonly involves the OBLIQUE RIDGE OF THE FIRST MAXILLARY MOLAR. Since the premature contact involves a supporting cusp tip (the distobuccal cusp of the mandibular first molar), it is recommended that the oblique ridge of the maxillary molar be adjusted to provide bilateral contacts.

Figure 5.2
(a) Diagrammatic arrangement of molar tooth contact with the jaw guided into RP. Note contact on maxillary lingual cusps (buccal inclines) and mandibular buccal cusps (lingual inclines) associated with the jaw position being more retruded. The arch form of the jaw does not coincide with maxillary arch form.

(b) Diagrammatic arrangements of molar teeth contact in IP. The arch forms of maxillary and mandibular teeth coincide and stable tooth contacts for jaw support result

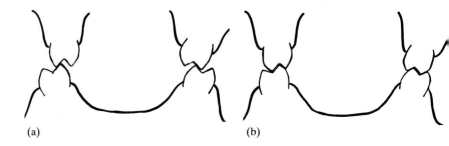

(a)   (b)

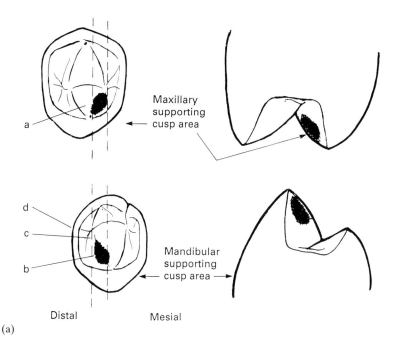

Maxillary supporting cusp area

a

d
c
b

Mandibular supporting cusp area

Distal   Mesial

(a)

Figure 5.3
(a) Diagrammatic representation of commonly occurring tooth contacts on maxillary and mandibular bicuspid teeth in RP accompanying tooth guidance. a. represents RP supracontact on maxillary supporting cusp on tooth 2.4; b. represents RP supracontact on mandibular supporting cusp on tooth 4.4; c. represents base of triangular ridge near central groove; d. represents marginal ridge area.
(b) Lateral view of jaw displacement from IP to RP. The contacts along cuspal inclines may be seen to be interferences along the final closing path into IP, in some instances. This pattern of cusp slope contact arises because of the retruded position of the lower arch which does not match the upper arch in RP as it does in IP. Compare Figure 5.2

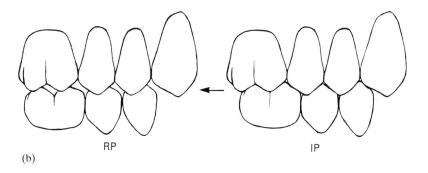

RP   IP

(b)

(iii) Another common site involves the bicuspids. Because of their position in the arch, premature contacts often involve the MESIOLINGUAL CUSP RIDGE OF THE FIRST MAXILLARY BICUSPID and the DISTAL CUSP RIDGE OF THE MANDIBULAR CANINE. This is most common in a Class II jaw relationship.

(iv) A premature contact may also be located along the DISTAL SLOPE OF THE TRIANGULAR RIDGE OF THE MANDIBULAR BICUSPID (Figure 5.3(a)), and the premature contact on the MAXILLARY BICUSPID would then be located on the MESIAL INCLINE OF THE TRIANGULAR RIDGE (see a). The premature contact shown in Figure 5.3(a) is high toward the cusp tip of the mandibular bicuspid (see b) and the end of the slide may be in the distal fossa (see c) or on the distal marginal ridge (see d).

Figure 5.4

(a) Diagrammatic representation of correct adjustment should it be necessary to reduce supporting cusp. The reduction should be primarily along the slope of the triangular or accessory ridge, rather than reducing cusp height unnecessarily.

(b) Diagrammatic representation of incorrect adjustment of cuspal edge that should be avoided with correct treatment planning and assessment of study casts

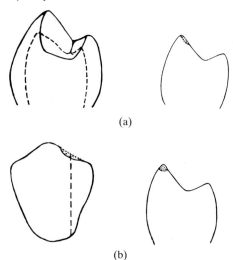

(a)

(b)

In Figure 5.3(a) the cusp tip and the distal cusp ridge of the mandibular bicuspid might be undermined or removed if it was adjusted; the cusp tip of the bicuspid is a supporting cusp and the distal cusp ridge is a functional ridge in laterotrusion. Thus the preferred adjustment (Figure 5.3(a)) should involve the maxillary bicuspids. Adjustment of the mandibular bicuspids, in the relationship shown, should only be considered where the adjustment of the maxillary bicuspids would result in excessive removal of tooth structure (Figure 5.4). Thus, the adjustment would be carried out first on the maxillary bicuspid and then, only if necessary, on the mandibular bicuspid.

In order to determine the preferred area of tooth adjustment, it is necessary to consider the following procedures on articulated study casts. This specific information may then be followed when the clinical occlusal adjustment is carried out:

– Evaluate the quality of the IP contacts, i.e. whether they are present on an area of tooth (e.g. marginal ridge), which would lead to stability, or on a cuspal incline, which would tend to instability;
– Identify and preserve:
  – IP or 'centric' contacts
  – supporting cusps;
– Eliminate unstable premature contacts on inclined planes.

3. Completion of adjustment
(a) Completion of RP adjustment
Contact vertical dimension at RP should be the same bilaterally. It may be similar at IP at the incisors or at the incisal pin of the articulator. If the incisal pin is set in contact with the incisal table in IP, the pin will be above the table in RP at a distance magnified by the arc of rotation of the jaw around the intercondylar axis, and the distance from the axis of rotation indicating the presence of a slide. THE SLIDE NEED NOT BE

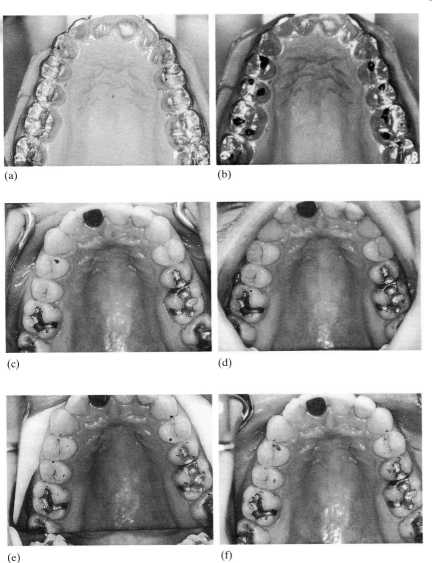

(a)

(b)

(c)

(d)

(e)

(f)

Figure 5.5 Occlusal adjustment.

(a) Maxillary study cast articulated and teeth coated with Tru-Fit lacquer for occlusal adjustment of casts.

(b) Maxillary study cast showing the completed adjustment. Areas of cuspal incline or marginal ridge which have been adjusted are coloured for clarity. The degree of adjustment required to achieve the desirable results, as described in text, can be seen to involve minimal reduction of tooth contour.

(c) Intra-oral view of maxillary arch indicating RP supracontacts on teeth 1.4 and 1.6.

(d) Intra-oral view of maxillary arch during RP adjustment; an increase in bilateral distribution of occlusal stops (black marks from GHM tape) is seen, but the adjustment is not yet complete.

(e) Intra-oral view of maxillary arch following the completion of the RP adjustment. Note the improved distribution of supporting stops (black marks from GHM foil) bilaterally and compare with pre-treatment situation in (c).

(f) Intra-oral view of maxillary arch following completion of both RP and MOP adjustment. Note the improved distribution of RP stops (as in (e)) and associated MOP stops (appearing as a lighter contact mark)

ELIMINATED, PROVIDED that the contacts are bilateral and are mesially directed.

(b) Completion of working side or laterotrusive adjustment

Working side adjustment is completed when the maxillary teeth relate in a lateral and lateral-protrusive direction to the mandibular teeth without interference, that is, a smooth uninterrupted glide outward to an edge-to-edge relationship of buccal cusps, and on return to RP and IP.

Only a small amount of the lingual inclines of the buccal cusps of the maxillary teeth may be removed to make multiple contacts in laterotrusion on casts. Where adequate canine overbite allows canine guidance, there may be no adjustment required.

(c) Completion of non-working side or mediotrusive adjustment
Non-working side adjustment is considered to be completed on casts when interferences to smooth gliding lateral movements from RP and IP have been eliminated. If necessary, a maxillary lingual cusp IP stop may be removed if it is involved as a balancing interference, but the lingual cusp should not be excessively reduced.

(d) Completion of protrusive adjustment
The protrusive adjustment is completed when all interferences to smooth gliding have been removed. All contact guidance should be on the maxillary cuspids and incisors. Adjustment of lingual aspects of the maxillary incisors should be limited to very moderate reduction, since the major consideration for adjusting this area is based on an evaluation of the patient. Only rarely is adjustment to lower anterior teeth indicated.

(e) Summary of procedures
1 Verification of mounting
2 Materials used:
2.1 Tru-fit die spacer (Taub Products*) or lacquer to cover contacting surfaces of teeth;
2.2 GHM tape† to mark tooth contacts;
2.3 Shim stock (Artus‡; Ivoclar§) to test the quality of tooth contacts.
3 Sequence:
3.1 RP adjustment to provide bilateral contacts on bicuspid and molar teeth;
3.2 RP–IP slide maintained with bilateral contact guidance on mesial inclines;
3.3 Non-working interferences eliminated to allow laterotrusive guidance on canines (CANINE GUIDANCE) or canines and bicuspids, and sometimes molar teeth as well (GROUP FUNCTION);
3.4 Protrusive guidance adjustment allowing canines and incisors to provide guidance.
4 Areas of tooth adjustment:
4.1 This should be restricted to the regions between the cusps, unless a cross-bite relationship will not allow this;
4.2 Preserve supporting cusp tips and recontour cuspal inclines, opposing fossae or marginal ridges, to provide cusp tip to fossae or marginal ridge contacts;
CAUTION: MINIMUM TOOTH ADJUSTMENT IS ESSENTIAL.

5.8 Clinical procedures

1. The principles of MINIMAL TOOTH REDUCTION described in Figures 5.1 to 5.4 are to be followed when carrying out an adjustment of natural teeth. Having already carefully adjusted the articulated study casts,

*Taub Products and Fusion Inc., Jersey City, NJ 07307, USA.
†Gebr. Hanel-Medizinal, D7440 Nürtingen, Germany.
‡Artus Corporation, Englewood, NJ 07631, USA.
§Ivoclar/Vivadent, Schaan FL9494, Liechtenstein.

it is a relatively easy task to follow this pattern of adjustment when commencing the adjustment of natural teeth. In this way clinical time is reduced, as the decisions concerning the most appropriate areas of teeth to be adjusted have already been made.

As well as initial assistance to the operator, articulated study casts are also valuable to be able to clearly illustrate to the patient:

(a) what teeth are to be adjusted;

(b) why this is necessary;

(c) the amount of adjustment required.

This latter aspect may well be of major importance in one's defence should dentolegal problems arise.

2. Summary of procedures

(a) Materials and instrumentation:
   - GHM tape to mark tooth contacts accurately
   - Miller holders* to support GHM tape
   - Shim stock – Artus or Ivoclar – to test the quality or degree of tooth contact
   - Cotton rolls to help to control saliva wetting the teeth
   - Composite finishing diamond (– FG and pear shaped: Star† WM2XF ISO Diamant‡ 830/022F) to adjust tooth surfaces
   - Air turbine (variable speed) for fine diamonds and red band micro-motor for polishing tooth surfaces
   - Polishing points – Deduco§, Shofu**
   - High velocity suction and air:water spray
   - Topical fluoride solution.

(b) Clinical sequence

1. Initial adjustment of teeth follows the adjustment of study casts.

2. RP adjustment to provide BILATERAL STOPS ON MESIALLY DIRECTED INCLINES OF SUPPORTING CUSPS. This may reduce the slide from RP to IP. However it is NOT necessary to remove the vertical component of the slide in order to provide a horizontal slide movement only.

3. Mediotrusive or non-working interferences adjusted to allow laterotrusive guidance on canines, or canines and bicuspid teeth.

4. Protrusive interferences adjusted to provide guidance on canines, or canine and incisor teeth.

5. Areas of tooth adjustment (as for pre-clinical procedures)
   - adjust region between cusps where possible
   - preserve supporting cusp tips and adjust cuspal inclines and marginal ridges to provide cusp-fossa or cusp-marginal ridge contacts.

6. MINIMUM TOOTH REDUCTION IS ESSENTIAL.

7. POLISH ALL ADJUSTED TOOTH SURFACES and APPLY TOPICAL FLUORIDE.

*Bausch Dental Co., D5000 Cologne 60, Germany.
†Star Dental Manufacturing Co. Inc, Valley Forge, Pa 19482, USA.
‡Iso Diamant, D8000 Munich, Germany.
§Deduco International Inc, Long Eddy, NY 12760, USA.
**Shofu Dental Manufacturing Co. Ltd, Kyoto, Japan.

References

Bailey, J. O. and Rugh, J. D. (1980) Effect of occlusal adjustment on bruxism as monitored by nocturnal emg recordings. *Journal of Dental Research,* **59** (Special Issue A): 317

Bakke, M., Møller, E. and Thorsen, N. M. (1980) Occlusal contact and maximal muscle activity in natural mandibular positions. *Journal of Dental Research,* **59** (Special Issue B): 892

Bakke, M., Møller, E. and Thorsen, N. M. (1982) Occlusal control of temporalis and masseter activity during mastication. *Journal of Dental Research,* **61** (Special Issue): 257

Barghi, N., Rugh, J. D. and Drago, C. J. (1979) Experimentally induced occlusal dysharmonies, nocturnal bruxism and MPD. *Journal of Dental Research,* **58** (Special Issue A): 317

Beyron, H. (1954) Occlusal changes in adult dentition. *Journal of the American Dental Association,* **48**, 674–686

Clark, G. T. and Adler, R. C. (1985) A critical evaluation of occlusal therapy: Occlusal adjustment procedures. *Journal of the American Dental Association,* **110**, 743–750

Dawson, P. E. (1989) *Evaluation, Diagnosis and Treatment of Occlusal Problems.* C. V. Mosby, St Louis, pp. 434–456

Forssell, H., Kirveskari, P. and Kangasniemi, P. (1986) Effect of occlusal adjustment on mandibular dysfunction. A double blind study. *Acta Odontologica Scandinavica,* **44**, 63–69

Forssell, H., Kirveskari, P. and Kangasniemi, P. (1987) Response to occlusal treatment in headache patients previously treated by mock occlusal adjustment. *Acta Odontologica Scandinavica,* **45**, 77–80

Goodman, P., Greene, C. and Laskin, D. (1976) Response of patients with myofascial pain dysfunction syndrome to mock equilibration. *Journal of the American Dental Association,* **92**, 755–758

Ingervall, B. and Hedegård, B. (1974) Subjective evaluation of functional disturbances of the masticatory system in young Swedish men. *Community Dentistry and Oral Epidemiology,* **2**, 149–152

Lund, J. P. and Widmer, C. G. (1989) An evaluation of the use of surface electromyography in the diagnosis, documentation and treatment of dental patients. *Journal of Craniomandibular Disorders Facial and Oral Pain,* **3**, 125–137

McCollum, B. B. (1955) Considering the mouth as a functioning unit as the basis of a dental diagnosis. In *A Research Report* (eds B. B. McCollum and C. E. Stuart), Scientific Press, Ventura

MacDonald, J. W. C. and Hannam, A. G. (1984) Relationship between occlusal contacts and jaw-closing muscle activity during tooth clenching. *Journal of Prosthetic Dentistry,* **52**, Part I: 718–729, Part II: 862–867

McNamara, D. C. (1976) Pathophysiology of occlusal balance. *Australian Dental Journal,* **21**, 247–251

McNamara, D. C. (1977) Occlusal adjustment for a physiologically balanced occlusion. *Journal of Prosthetic Dentistry,* **38**, 284–293

Mann, A. W. and Pankey, L. D. (1963) The PM philosophy of occlusal rehabilitation. *Dental Clinics of North America,* 621–638

Manns, A., Chan, C. and Miralles, R. (1987) Influence of group function and canine guidance on electromyographic activity of elevator muscles. *Journal of Prosthetic Dentistry,* **57**, 494–501

Marbach, J. J. (1976) Phantom bite. *American Journal of Orthodontics,* **70**, 190–199

Marbach, J. J. (1978) Phantom bite syndrome. *American Journal of Psychiatry,* **135**, 476–479

Marbach, J. J., Varoscak, J. R., Blank, R. T. and Lund, P. (1983) 'Phantom bite': Classification and treatment. *Journal of Prosthetic Dentistry,* **49**, 556–559

Matthews, B. (1975) Mastication. In *Applied Physiology of the Mouth* (ed. C. L. B. Lavelle), John Wright, Bristol, pp. 199–242

Moozeh, M. B., Suit, S. R. and Bissada, N. F. (1981) Tooth mobility measurements following two methods of eliminating non-working side occlusal interferences. *Journal of Clinical Periodontology,* **8**, 424–430

Munro, A. (1978) Monosymptomatic hypochondriacal psychosis. *Canadian Psychiatric Association Journal,* **23**, 497–500

Nielsen, I. L., Marcel, T., Chun, D. and Miller, A. J. (1990) Patterns of mandibular movement in subjects with craniomandibular disorders. *Journal of Prosthetic Dentistry,* **63**, 202–217

Ramfjord, S. P. (1961) Bruxism, a clinical and electromyographic study. *Journal of the American Dental Association,* **62**, 21–44

Ramfjord, S. P. and Ash, M. M. (1983) *Occlusion*, 3rd edn, Ch. 13, W. B. Saunders, Philadelphia, pp. 384–424

Schuyler, C. H. (1935) Fundamental principles in the correction of occlusal dysharmony, natural and artificial. *Journal of the American Dental Association,* **22**, 1193–1202

Sheikholeslam, A., Møller, E. and Lous, I. (1982) Postural and maximal activity in elevators of mandible before and after treatment of functional disorders. *Scandinavian Journal of Dental Research,* **90**, 37–46

Sherman, R. A. (1985) Relationships between jaw pain and jaw muscle contraction level: underlying factors and treatment effectiveness. *Journal of Prosthetic Dentistry,* **54**, 114–118

Sternbach, R. A. (1974) *Pain Patients Traits and Treatment*, Academic Press, New York, pp. 5–11

Stuart, C. E. and Stallard, H. (1960) Principles involved in restoring occlusion to natural teeth. *Journal of Prosthetic Dentistry,* **10**, 304–313

Yemm, R. (1979) Neurophysiologic studies of temporomandibular joint dysfunction. In *Temporomandibular Joint Function and Dysfunction* (eds G. A. Zarb and G. E. Carlsson), Munksgaard, Copenhagen, pp. 215–237

Terminology

1. Pain

A list with definitions and notes on usage

Abstracted from *Pain* 1986; Suppl. 3: 5216–5221. The information originally appeared in a less comprehensive form in *Pain* 1979; **6**: 249–252.

The use of individual terms often varies widely. That need not be a cause of distress provided that each author makes clear precisely how he employs a word. Nevertheless, it is convenient and helpful to others if words can be used which have agreed technical meanings. Following correspondence and meetings during the period 1976–1978, the present committee agreed on the definitions which follow and the notes have been prepared by the chairman in the light of members' comments. The definitions are intended to be specific and explanatory and to serve as an operational framework, not as a constraint on future development. They represent agreement between diverse specialities including anaesthesiology, dentistry, neurology, neurosurgery, neurophysiology, psychiatry and psychology. A starting point for some of these definitions was provided by the reports of a workshop on Orofacial Pain held at the US National Institute of Dental Research in November, 1974.

The terms and definitions are not meant to provide a comprehensive glossary but rather a minimum standard vocabulary for members of different disciplines who work in the field of pain. We hope that they will prove acceptable to all those in the health professions who deal with pain. Not only are they a limited selection from available terms, but except for pain itself, terms are defined primarily in relation to the skin and the special senses are excluded. They may be used when appropriate for responses to somatic stimulation elsewhere or to the viscera. Except for Pain, the arrangement is in alphabetical order.

It is important to emphasize something that was implicit in the previous definitions, but was not specifically stated, that is that the terms have been developed for use in clinical practice rather than for experimental work, physiology, or anatomical purposes.

Pain

An unpleasant sensory and emotional experience associated with actual or potential tissue damage, or described in terms of such damage.

Note: Pain is always subjective. Each individual learns the application of the word through experiences related to injury in early life. Biologists recognize that those stimuli which cause pain are liable to damage tissue. Accordingly, pain is that experience which we associate with actual or potential tissue damage. It is unquestionably a sensation in a part or parts of the body, but it is also always unpleasant and therefore also an emotional experience. Experiences which resemble pain, e.g. pricking, but are not unpleasant, should not be called pain. Unpleasant abnormal experiences (dysaesthesiae q.v.) may also be pain but are not necessarily so because, subjectively, they may not have the usual sensory qualities of pain.

Many people report pain in the absence of tissue damage or any likely pathophysiological cause and usually this happens for psychological reasons. There is usually no way to distinguish their experience from that due to tissue damage if we take the subjective report. If they regard their experience as pain and if they report it in the same way as pain caused by tissue damage, it should be accepted as pain. This definition avoids tying pain to the stimulus. Activity induced in the nociceptor and nociceptive pathways by a noxious stimulus is not pain, which is always a psychological state, even though we may well appreciate that pain most often has a proximate physical cause.

Allodynia

Pain due to a stimulus which does not normally provoke pain.

Note: This was first introduced as a term intended to refer to the situation where otherwise normal tissues, which may have abnormal innervation or may be referral sites for other loci, give rise to pain on stimulation by non-noxious means.

In the original definition the words 'to normal skin' were used and later were omitted in order to remove any suggestion that allodynia applied only to referred pain. Originally, also, the pain-provoking stimulus was described as 'non-noxious'. However, a stimulus may be noxious at some times and not at others, for example, with intact skin and sunburned skin, and also, the boundaries of noxious stimulation may be hard to delineate. Since the Committee aimed at providing terms for clinical use, it did not wish to define them by reference to the specific physical characteristics of the stimulation, e.g. pressure in kilopascals per square centimetre, etc. Moreover, even in intact skin there is little evidence one way or the other that a strong painful pinch to a normal person does or does not damage tissue.

Accordingly, it was considered to be preferable to define allodynia in terms of the response to clinical stimuli and to point out that the normal response to the stimulus could always be tested elsewhere in the body, usually in a corresponding part.

It is important to recognize that allodynia involves a change in the quality of a sensation, whether tactile, thermal, or of any other sort. The original modality is normally non-painful but the response is painful. There is thus a loss of specificity of a sensory modality. By contrast, hyperalgesia (q.v.) represents an augmented response in a specific mode, viz. pain. With other cutaneous modalities, hyperaesthesia is the term which corresponds to hyperalgesia and as with hyperalgesia, the quality is not altered. In allodynia the stimulus mode and the response mode differ, unlike the situation with hyperalgesia. This distinction should not be confused by the fact that allodynia and hyperalgesia can be plotted with overlap along the same continuum of physical intensity in certain circumstances, for example, with pressure or temperature.

See also the notes on hyperalgesia and hyperpathia.

Anaesthesia dolorosa

Pain in an area or region which is anaesthetic.

Analgesia

Absence of pain in response to stimulation which would normally be painful.

Note: As with allodynia (q.v.) the stimulus is defined by its usual subjective effects.

Causalgia

A syndrome of sustained burning pain, allodynia, and hyperpathia after a traumatic nerve lesion, often combined with vasomotor and sudomotor dysfunction and later trophic changes.

Central pain

Pain associated with a lesion of the central nervous system.

Dysaesthesia

An unpleasant abnormal sensation, whether spontaneous or evoked.

Note: Compare with pain and with paraesthesia. Special cases of dysaesthesia include hyperalgesia and allodynia. A dysaesthesia should always be unpleasant and a paraesthesia should not be unpleasant, although it is recognized that the borderline may present some difficulties when it comes to deciding as to whether a sensation is pleasant or unpleasant. It should always be specified whether the sensations are spontaneous or evoked.

Hyperaesthesia

Increased sensitivity to stimulation, excluding the special senses.

Note: The stimulus and locus should be specified. Hyperaesthesia may refer to various modes of cutaneous sensibility including touch and thermal sensation without pain, as well as to pain. The word is used to indicate both diminished threshold to any stimulus and an increased response to stimuli that are normally recognized.
Allodynia is suggested for pain after stimulation which is not normally painful. Hyperaesthesia includes both allodynia and hyperalgesia, but the more specific terms should be used wherever they are applicable.

Hyperalgesia

An increased response to a stimulus which is normally painful.

Note: The changes here relate to two matters. One is the avoidance of the word noxious in the definition, because of difficulties in its use. The second is the inclusion of some features of allodynia (q.v.) in the definition of hyperalgesia.

Many cases of hyperalgesia have features of allodynia. The term allodynia should be preferred when there is not an increased response to a stimulus which normally provokes pain. However, when there is also a response of increased pain to a stimulus which normally is painful, hyperalgesia is the appropriate word.

It should also be recognized that with allodynia the stimulus and the response are in different modes, whereas with hyperalgesia they are in the same mode.

See also notes on allodynia and hyperpathia.

Hyperpathia

A painful syndrome, characterized by increased reaction to a stimulus, especially a repetitive stimulus, as well as an increased threshold.

Note: It may occur with hyperaesthesia, hyperalgesia, or dysaesthesia. Faulty identification and localization of the stimulus, delay, radiating sensation, and after-sensation may be present, and the pain is often explosive in character. The change in this note is the inclusion of hyperalgesia explicitly, whereas previously it was implied, since hyperaesthesia was mentioned and hyperalgesia is a special case of hyperaesthesia.

The implications of some of the above definitions may be summarized for convenience as follows:

allodynia:	lowered threshold:	stimulus and response mode differ
hyperalgesia:	increased response:	stimulus and response mode are the same
hyperpathia:	raised threshold: increased response:	stimulus and response may be the same or different
hypoalgesia: (see below)	raised threshold: lower response:	stimulus and response mode are the same

The above essentials of the definitions do not have to be symmetrical at present. Lowered threshold may occur with hyperalgesia but is not required. Also, there is no category for lowered threshold and lowered response – if it ever occurs.

Hypoaesthesia

Decreased sensitivity to stimulation, excluding the special senses.

Note: Stimulation and locus to be specified.

Hypoalgesia

Diminished pain in response to a normally painful stimulus.

Note: Hypoalgesia was formerly defined as diminished sensitivity to noxious stimulation, making it a particular case of hypoaesthesia (q.v.).

However, it now refers only to the occurrence of relatively less pain in response to stimulation that produces pain. Hypoaesthesia covers the case of diminished sensitivity to stimulation that is normally painful.

Neuralgia

Pain in the distribution of a nerve or nerves.

Note: Common usage, especially in Europe, often implies a paroxysmal quality, but neuralgia should not be reserved for paroxysmal pains.

Neuritis

Inflammation of a nerve or nerves.

Note: Not to be used unless inflammation is thought to be present.

Neuropathy

A disturbance of function or pathological change in a nerve:
in one nerve – mononeuropathy;
in several nerves – mononeuropathy multiplex;
if diffuse and bilateral – polyneuropathy.

Note: Neuritis is a special case of neuropathy and is now reserved for inflammatory processes affecting nerves. Neuropathy is not intended to cover cases like neurapraxis, neurotmesis, or section of a nerve.

Nociceptor

A receptor preferentially sensitive to a noxious stimulus or to a stimulus which would become noxious if prolonged.

NOTE: AVOID USE OF TERMS LIKE PAIN RECEPTOR OR PAIN PATHWAY.

Noxious stimulus

A noxious stimulus is one which is damaging to normal tissues.

Note: Although the definition of a noxious stimulus has been retained, the term is not used in this list to define other terms.

Pain threshold

The least experience of pain which a subject can recognize.

Note: Traditionally the threshold has often been defined, as we defined it formerly, as the least stimulus intensity at which a subject perceives pain. Properly defined the threshold is really the experience of the patient, whereas the intensity measured is an external event. It has been common usage for most pain research workers to define the threshold in terms of the stimulus and that should be avoided. However, the threshold stimulus can be recognized as such and measured. In psychophysics, thresholds are defined as the level at which 50% of stimuli are recognized.

In that case, the pain threshold would be the level at 50% of stimuli would be recognized as painful. The stimulus is not pain (q.v.) and cannot be a measure of pain.

Pain tolerance level

The greatest level of pain which a subject is prepared to tolerate.

Note: As with pain threshold, the pain tolerance level is the subjective experience of the individual. The stimuli which are normally measured in relation to its production are the pain tolerance level stimuli and not the level itself. Thus, the same argument applies to pain tolerance level as to pain threshold and it is not defined in terms of the external stimulation as such.

Paraesthesia

An abnormal sensation, whether spontaneous or evoked.

Note: Compare with dysaesthesia. It has been agreed to recommend that paraesthesia be used to describe an abnormal sensation which is not unpleasant whilst dysaesthesia be used preferentially for an abnormal sensation which is considered to be unpleasant. The use of one term (paraesthesia) to indicate spontaneous sensations and the other to refer to evoked sensations is not favoured.

There is a sense in which, since paraesthesia refers to abnormal sensations in general, it might include dysaesthesia but the reverse is not true. Dysaesthesia does not include all abnormal sensations, but only those which are unpleasant.

2. Headache

Headache has recently been assessed and a classification and diagnostic criteria have been defined for headache disorders, cranial neuralgias and facial pain.

This has been published as a special supplement in *Cephalgia* 1988; **8** (Suppl. 7): 1–96.

The classification is listed below as an indication of the extent of headache and the need to consider the patient's symptoms and clinical signs within a broad framework for differential diagnosis.

Section 2 classifies tension-type headache either associated with pericranial muscles or not and in this context jaw and cervical muscles may contribute to tension headache with pain referral.

Section 11 classifies headache associated with specific facial structures including skull, neck, eyes, ears, nose and sinuses, teeth and jaws, and the TM joints. It is this area where the dental clinician has a specific responsibility. Differential diagnosis must critically consider these areas and referral to specialist dental or medical clinicians may be indicated in the absence of a specific diagnosis being made.

The importance of making a specific diagnosis to allow for a specific treatment sequence cannot be over-emphasized. It must also be appreciated that many patients have more than one headache. It is not uncommon for patients to present with migraine together with tension headache and craniomandibular pain involving jaw muscles and TM joints. Also, patients presenting with craniomandibular pain and dysfunction involving jaw muscles, TM joints and cervical muscles and joints are not uncommon.

It will be appreciated that this classification will alert all clinicians to the need to consider the presence of, and hopefully identify, specific headaches and pain problems occurring together.

Classification

Taken from *Cephalgia* 1988; **8** (Suppl. 7): 1–96.

1 Migraine
1.1 Migraine without aura
1.2 Migraine with aura
    1.2.1 Migraine with typical aura
    1.2.2 Migraine with prolonged aura
    1.2.3 Familial hemiplegic migraine
    1.2.4 Basilar migraine
    1.2.5 Migraine aura without headache
    1.2.6 Migraine with acute onset aura
1.3 Ophthalmoplegic migraine
1.4 Retinal migraine
1.5 Childhood periodic syndromes that may be precursors to or associated with migraine
    1.5.1 Benign paroxysmal vertigo of childhood
    1.5.2 Alternating hemiplegia of childhood
1.6 Complications of migraine
    1.6.1 Status migrainosus
    1.6.2 Migrainous infarction
1.7 Migrainous disorder not fulfilling above criteria

2 Tension-type headaches
2.1 Episodic tension-type headache
    2.1.1 Episodic tension-type headache associated with disorder of pericranial muscles
    2.1.2 Episodic tension-type headache unassociated with disorder of pericranial muscles
2.2 Chronic tension-type headache
    2.2.1 Chronic tension-type headache associated with disorder of pericranial muscles

2.2.2 Chronic tension-type headache unassociated with disorder of
pericranial muscles
2.3 Headache of the tension-type not fulfilling above criteria

3 Cluster headache and chronic paroxysmal hemicrania
3.1 Cluster headache
    3.1.1 Cluster headache periodicity undetermined
    3.1.2 Episodic cluster headache
    3.1.3 Chronic cluster headache
        3.1.3.1 Unremitting from onset
        3.1.3.2 Evolved from episodic
3.2 Chronic paroxysmal hemicrania
3.3 Cluster headache-like disorder not fulfilling above criteria

4 Miscellaneous headaches unassociated with structural lesion
4.1 Idiopathic stabbing headache
4.2 External compression headache
4.3 Cold stimulus headache
    4.3.1 External application of a cold stimulus
    4.3.2 Ingestion of a cold stimulus
4.4 Benign cough headache
4.5 Benign exertional headache
4.6 Headache associated with sexual activity
    4.6.1 Dull type
    4.6.2 Explosive type
    4.6.3 Postural type

5 Headache associated with head trauma
5.1 Acute post-traumatic headache
    5.1.1 With significant head trauma and/or confirmatory signs
    5.1.2 With minor head trauma and no confirmatory signs
5.2 Chronic post-traumatic headache
    5.2.1 With significant head trauma and/or confirmatory signs
    5.2.2 With minor head trauma and no confirmatory signs

6 Headache associated with vascular disorders
6.1 Acute ischaemic cerebrovascular disease
    6.1.1 Transient ischaemic attack (TIA)
    6.1.2 Thromboembolic stroke
6.2 Intracranial haematoma
    6.2.1 Intracerebral haematoma
    6.2.2 Subdural haematoma
    6.2.3 Epidural haematoma
6.3 Subarachnoid haemorrhage
6.4 Unruptured vascular malformation
    6.4.1 Arteriovenous malformation
    6.4.2 Saccular aneurism
6.5 Arteritis
    6.5.1 Giant-cell arteritis
    6.5.2 Other systemic arteritides
    6.5.3 Primary intracranial arteritis

6.6 Carotid or vertebral artery pain
    6.6.1 Carotid or vertebral dissection
    6.6.2 Carotidynia (idiopathic)
    6.6.3 Post-endarterectomy headache
6.7 Venous thrombosis
6.8 Arterial hypertension
    6.8.1 Acute pressor response to exogenous agent
    6.8.2 Phaeochromocytoma
    6.8.3 Malignant (accelerated) hypertension
    6.8.4 Pre-eclampsia and eclampsia
6.9 Headache associated with other vascular disorder

7 Headache associated with non-vascular intracranial disorder
7.1 High cerebrospinal fluid pressure
    7.1.1 Benign intracranial hypertension
    7.1.2 High pressure hydrocephalus
7.2 Low cerebrospinal fluid pressure
    7.2.1 Post-lumbar puncture headache
    7.2.2 Cerebrospinal fluid fistula headache
7.3 Intracranial infection
7.4 Intracranial sarcoidosis and other non-infectious inflammatory diseases
7.5 Headache related to intrathecal injections
    7.5.1 Direct effect
    7.5.2 Due to chemical meningitis
7.6 Intracranial neoplasm
7.7 Headache associated with other intracranial disorder

8 Headache associated with substances or their withdrawal
8.1 Headache induced by acute substance use or exposure
    8.1.1 Nitrate/nitrite induced headache
    8.1.2 Monosodium glutamate induced headache
    8.1.3 Carbon monoxide induced headache
    8.1.4 Alcohol induced headache
    8.1.5 Other substances
8.2 Headache induced by chronic substance use or exposure
    8.2.1 Ergotamine induced headache
    8.2.2 Analgesics abuse headache
    8.2.3 Other substances
8.3 Headache from substance withdrawal (acute use)
    8.3.1 Alcohol withdrawal headache (hangover)
    8.3.2 Other substances
8.4 Headache from substance withdrawal (chronic use)
    8.4.1 Ergotamine withdrawal headache
    8.4.2 Caffeine withdrawal headache
    8.4.3 Narcotics abstinence headache
    8.4.4 Other substances
8.5 Headache associated with substances but with uncertain mechanism
    8.5.1 Birth control pills or oestrogens
    8.5.2 Other substances

9 Headache associated with non-cephalic infection
9.1 Viral infection
    9.1.1 Focal non-cephalic
    9.1.2 Systemic
9.2 Bacterial infection
    9.2.1 Focal non-cephalic
    9.2.2 Systemic (septicemia)
9.3 Headache related to other infection

10 Headache associated with metabolic disorder
10.1 Hypoxia
    10.1.1 High altitude headache
    10.1.2 Hypoxic headache
    10.1.3 Sleep apnoea headache
10.2 Hypercapnia
10.3 Mixed hypoxia and hypercapnia
10.4 Hypoglycaemia
10.5 Dialysis
10.6 Headache related to other metabolic abnormality

11 Headache or facial pain associated with disorder of cranium, neck, eyes, ears, nose sinuses, teeth, mouth or other facial or cranial structures
11.1 Cranial bone
11.2 Neck
    11.2.1 Cervical spine
    11.2.2 Retropharyngeal tendonitis
11.3 Eyes
    11.3.1 Acute glaucoma
    11.3.2 Refractive errors
    11.3.3 Heterophoria or heterotopia
11.4 Ears
11.5 Nose and sinuses
    11.5.1 Acute sinus headache
    11.5.2 Other diseases of nose or sinuses
11.6 Teeth, jaws and related structures
11.7 Temporomandibular joint disease

12 Cranial neuralgias, nerve trunk pain and deafferentation pain
12.1 Persistent (in contrast to tic-like) pain of cranial nerve origin
    12.1.1 Compression or distortion of cranial nerves and second or third cervical roots
    12.1.2 Demyelination of cranial nerves
        12.1.2.1 Optic neuritis (retrobulbar neuritis)
    12.1.3 Infarction of cranial nerves
        12.1.3.1 Diabetic neuritis
    12.1.4 Inflammation of cranial nerves
        12.1.4.1 Herpes zoster
        12.1.4.2 Chronic post-herpetic neuralgia
    12.1.5 Tolosa–Hunt syndrome

Clinical health questionnaires

UNIVERSITY OF SYDNEY
DEPARTMENT OF PROSTHETIC DENTISTRY

CLINICAL HEALTH QUESTIONNAIRE
NO. 1: GENERAL INFORMATION

The main concerns of the Clinic are to understand your problem and to help you by providing the best treatment possible. Most people referred to this Clinic have complex or difficult dental problems. In order to understand each patient's problem, an extensive case history is needed. Please fill in the answers to this questionnaire as fully as you can and bring it with you to your first appointment. Not every question may be applicable to your particular problem. If you have difficulty in answering any question, leave it out and discuss it with your dentist at your first consultation.

What are your main symptoms? _____

_____

What dental or medical treatment have you already had for these symptoms?

_____
_____
_____

Did any of these treatments help   YES   NO   DO NOT KNOW
your symptoms?

   If "yes" which ones helped? _____

Did any of these treatments make   YES   NO   DO NOT KNOW
your symptoms worse?

   If "yes" which ones made you worse?

_____
_____

When did your symptoms first appear?

_____
_____

What do you think is the main cause of your symptoms?

_____
_____

Name and address of referring doctor/dentist

_____
_____
_____

Name and address of family doctor

_____
_____
_____

SURNAME: Mr. Ms. Dr. Sr.
           Mrs. Miss Rev. _____

OTHER NAMES: _____

ADDRESS: Home _____

           _____ Postcode _____

    Business _____

           _____ Postcode _____

TELEPHONE: Home _____ Business _____

          DATE OF BIRTH: _____

MARITAL STATUS: Married   Single   Divorced
                Widowed   Separated Other

COUNTRY OF BIRTH: _____

NUMBER OF YEARS IN AUSTRALIA: _____ years
                        PARTNER'S
OCCUPATION: _____ OCCUPATION _____

PREVIOUS OCCUPATION (if retired or
             doing home duties): _____

AT WHAT LEVEL DID YOU COMPLETE YOUR FORMAL EDUCATION

_____

Place a tick in the box next to any of the symptoms below which you have noticed yourself or which your family or friends have noticed.

*(1)	Pain in your face or jaw	☐	(17) Muscle tension	☐
*(2)	Pain in jaw joint	☐	(18) Grinding your teeth at night	☐
*(3)	Pain in your neck area	☐	(19) Clenching your teeth	☐
*(4)	Pain in your arm	☐	(20) Chewing or biting movements at times other than meal times	☐
*(5)	Headaches or earaches	☐	(21) Biting or sucking your cheeks, tongue or lips	☐
*(6)	Toothache or tooth sensitivity	☐	(22) Biting or sucking your fingernails, pens, pencils, etc.	☐
*(7)	Sore tongue or gums	☐	(23) Numbness in your face or mouth	☐
*(8)	Swollen jaw joint	☐	(24) Swelling in your face or mouth	☐
(9)	Noises in your ears	☐	(25) Nausea	☐
(10)	Blocked ears	☐	(26) Sinusitis	☐
(11)	Dizziness	☐	(27) Teeth chipping	☐
(12)	Difficulty in opening your mouth wide	☐	(28) Teeth wearing down	☐
(13)	Difficulty in closing your mouth after opening it wide	☐	(29) Inability to wear your dentures	☐
(14)	Locking of your jaw	☐	(30) Moving dentures about in your mouth with your tongue or by sucking	☐
(15)	Difficulty in chewing	☐		
(16)	Clicking in your jaw joint	☐	(31) Gagging	☐

Has there been any change in your general health in the last year?

YES   NO

Are you receiving treatment for a medical condition at present?

YES   NO

If "yes", what is the medical condition? _____

_____

What is the treatment? _____

_____

Please list any other operations, accidents or serious illness you have had:

Operations, accident or illness	Approximate date

Please list below the names and doses of all the medicines and tablets you are taking at present. Include any medicines or tablets you take only occasionally.

Name of medicine or tablets	Dose	Number of times per day

How often have you been to the dentist in the past?

6-monthly   annually   irregularly

☐   ☐   ☐

Do you wear dentures?   YES   NO

Please describe any special problem you have with your dentures:

_____

Please describe any special dental treatment you have had in the past e.g. orthodontic treatment (bands, appliances) root canal therapy, periodontal (gum) treatment, surgery, tooth extractions.

Special treatment	Approximate date

Do you smoke?   YES   NO

If "yes", less than 10 cigarettes a day?   ☐

between 10–20 cigarettes a day?   ☐

more than 20 cigarettes a day?   ☐

Do you drink alcoholic drinks?   YES   NO

If "yes", less than once a week?   ☐

between 2–5 glasses a week?   ☐

about 1–2 glasses a day?   ☐

more than 2 glasses a day?   ☐

Do you drink tea, coffee or coca-cola?   YES   NO

If "yes", how many cups per day?

tea? _____

coffee? _____

coca-cola? _____

Do you take regular physical exercise?   YES   NO

If "yes", please describe _____

_____

Are you experiencing stress in any area of your life at the present time?   YES   NO

If "yes" is your stress related to any of the following areas of life:

Marriage   Family   Work   Other

Finances   Bereavement   Health

Is there anything else you can tell us that would help us to understand your problem?

_____

_____

_____

_____

UNIVERSITY OF SYDNEY
DEPARTMENT OF PROSTHETIC DENTISTRY

Name ....

CLINICAL HEALTH QUESTIONNAIRE   NO 2 : PAIN

Date ....

We notice that you mentioned pain as one of your symptoms. Because pain is a very individual experience, not the same for everyone, could you please help us to understand what your pain is like by answering the following questions as fully as you can.

1.   <u>LOCATION</u>: Where is your pain located? On the drawings below mark or colour any area which is painful.

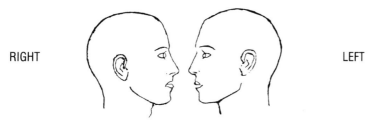

RIGHT   LEFT

2.   <u>SEVERITY</u>: The line below is a scale for pain ranging from no pain at all to the worst pain imaginable. Place a cross on this line to show us how severe your pain problem is most of the time.

No pain   Very severe pain

If your pain varies and is worse at some times than others, put a tick on the line to show us how bad it gets; and another tick at the point on the line to show us the least pain you experience.

If you have more than one pain (e.g. a headache and a jaw pain) and would find it easier to rate these separately, please do so on the scales below.

(1) Which pain are you rating? ....

No pain   Very severe pain

(2) Which pain are you rating? ....

No pain   Very severe pain

(3) Which pain are you rating? ....

No pain   Very severe pain

3.   <u>PAIN CORRELATES</u>: Have you noticed a relationship of any kind between your pain and any of the items listed below. Put a tick in the box.

Is your pain worse: after eating?
                       during meals?
                       in the mornings?
                       in the evenings?
                       during the night?
                       while talking?
                       while laughing?
                       or yawning?
                       when lying down?
                       when under mental stress?
                       when muscles are tense?
                       when cold?

Describe any other
relationship you
have noticed?   ....
                      ....

Please answer the questions on the back of this page

4. <u>PAIN DESCRIPTION</u>: Please underline any word below that could be used to describe your pain.

1	2	3	4	5
Flickering	Jumping	Pricking	Sharp	Pinching
Quivering	Flashing	Boring	Cutting	Pressing
Pulsing	Shooting	Drilling	Lacerating	Gnawing
Throbbing		Stabbing		Cramping
Beating		Lancinating		Crushing
Pounding				

6	7	8	9	10
Tugging	Hot	Tingling	Dull	Tender
Pulling	Burning	Itchy	Sore	Taut
Wrenching	Scalding	Smarting	Hurting	Rasping
	Searing	Stinging	Aching	Splitting

11	12	13	14	15
Tiring	Sickening	Fearful	Punishing	Wretched
Exhausting	Suffocating	Frightful	Gruelling	Binding
		Terrifying	Cruel	
			Vicious	
			Killing	

16	17	18	19	20
Annoying	Spreading	Tight	Cool	Nagging
Troublesome	Radiating	Numb	Cold	Nauseating
Miserable	Penetrating	Drawing	Freezing	Agonizing
Intense	Piercing	Squeezing		Dreadful
Unbearable		Tearing		Torturing

5. <u>PAIN DURATION</u>: When you have the pain, which of the words below best describe the time pattern of the pain? Underline any word that applies.

1	2	3
Continuous	Rhythmic	Brief
Steady	Periodic	Momentary
Constant	Intermittent	Transient

How often does the pain occur? Place a tick in the box next to the answer that best describes your pain.

- [ ] Only occasionally with no fixed pattern
- [ ] Occasionally, lasting for a day or more
- [ ] Frequently with no fixed pattern
- [ ] Frequently, lasting for a day or more
- [ ] Every day, with no fixed pattern
- [ ] Every day and seems related to certain times or things I do
- [ ] Every day and is always present

UNIVERSITY OF SYDNEY
DEPARTMENT OF PROSTHETIC DENTISTRY

CLINICAL HEALTH QUESTIONNAIRE   NO 3 : PAIN-TENSION DIARY

The aim of this diary is to provide information which will help us in diagnosis and treatment of your condition and help you to become aware of activities or circumstances affecting your condition. To keep the diary, please make a rating once each hour as follows. Note down your main activity for that hour and whether you were active or reclining. You need not fill in the columns while you are asleep. Just note the times you have been sleeping. In the medications column, record any medicines or tablets that you take, noting down the dosage (e.g. 30 mg) from the label on the bottle or packet.

If you are experiencing pain or discomfort of any kind, make a rating of your pain level each hour according to the scale below:

        0 = no pain at all
     1–4 = mild levels of pain
        5 = moderate levels of pain
     6–9 = more severe levels of pain
      10 = very severe pain.

Then, in the tension column, make a rating of your muscle tension for that hour, according to the scale below:

        0 = muscles relaxed, teeth apart
        1 = tightness of muscles but teeth still apart
        2 = tightness of muscles, teeth occasionally together
        3 = teeth together quite often
        4 = teeth together most of the time.

During meal-times, rate only muscle tension that occurs when you are NOT eating.

This diary, filled in over a period of 7 days, will enable us to see whether there is a pattern to your pain or your muscle tension. Sometimes we find that people habitually bite or clench their teeth together without being aware of it until they start to monitor their daily behaviour for the diary. Usually clenching occurs when you are tense or when you are concentrating on something else. You may not be aware of clenching during your sleep, however your spouse, family or friends may have noticed tooth clenching or grinding movements when you are sleeping. If so, please note down any information they are able to give you. You may notice other sensations or you may become aware of relationships between pain or tension and thoughts or feelings. Please note down anything that you think could be relevant to treatment or could help us to understand your dental problem.

SAMPLE
<u>DIARY</u>

TIME	SITTING OR MOVING	RECLINING	MEDICATION	PAIN	TENSION
MIDNIGHT 12–1		Sleep			
1–2		"			
2–3		"			
3–4		"			
4–5		"			
5–6		"			
6–7		Sleep	2 Panadeine mg	7	4
7–8	Shower, eat breakfast			7	3
8–9	Travel to work by car		2 Digesic	8	4
9–10	Paper work			3	1
10–11	Interview			4	1
11–12	Paperwork			3	1
MIDDAY 12–1	Paperwork			2	1
1–2	Lunch		1 Serepax 15 mg	5	2
2–3	Meeting		2 Panadeine	6	3
3–4	Meeting			7	3
4–5	Travel by car			8	4
5–6		Reading	2 Digesic	4	2
6–7	Helping kids with homework		1 Serepax	3	2
7–8	Drink, dinner			2	2
8–9	Washing up, kids to bed			1	2
9–10		Relax TV		1	1
10–11		Relax TV	1 Mogadon	0	1
11–12		Sleep			

UNIVERSITY OF SYDNEY
DEPARTMENT OF PROSTHETIC DENTISTRY

FOLLOW UP QUESTIONNAIRE

Name ....

Date ....

Your answers to these questions help us to have a clear understanding of how you are feeling and of any changes, for the better or the worse, in the symptoms you are experiencing. Please answer each question as fully as you can.

1. Please describe any problems or difficulties you have experienced with your treatment since your last visit.

_____

_____

2. Have you experienced any changes or stresses in your life which have made you feel more tense or less tense since your last appointment?

   YES   NO

   If yes, please describe briefly what has happened.

_____

_____

3. Place a tick in the box next to any of the symptoms below which you have noticed yourself or which your family or friends have noticed.

*(1) Pain in your face or jaw ☐	(17) Muscle tension ☐
*(2) Pain in jaw joint ☐	(18) Grinding your teeth at night ☐
*(3) Pain in your neck area ☐	(19) Clenching your teeth ☐
*(4) Pain in your arm ☐	(20) Chewing or biting movements at times other than meal times ☐
*(5) Headaches or earaches ☐	(21) Biting or sucking your cheeks, tongue or lips ☐
*(6) Toothache or tooth sensitivity ☐	(22) Biting or sucking your fingernails, pens, pencils, etc. ☐
*(7) Sore tongue or gums ☐	(23) Numbness in your face or mouth ☐
*(8) Swollen jaw joint ☐	(24) Swelling in your face or mouth ☐
(9) Noises in your ears ☐	(25) Nausea ☐
(10) Blocked ears ☐	(26) Sinusitis ☐
(11) Dizziness ☐	(27) Teeth chipping ☐
(12) Difficulty in opening your mouth wide ☐	(28) Teeth wearing down ☐
(13) Difficulty in closing your mouth after opening it wide ☐	(29) Inability to wear your dentures ☐
(14) Locking of your jaw ☐	(30) Moving dentures about in your mouth with your tongue or by sucking ☐
(15) Difficulty in chewing ☐	(31) Gagging ☐
(16) Clicking in your jaw joint ☐	

Isokinetic exercises — instructions to patients

ISOKINETIC EXERCISES

- INSTRUCTIONS TO PATIENTS

1. Seat yourself comfortably at a
    table.

2. Place your chin in the palm of your
    right hand with the elbow of the
    right arm resting on the table.

3. Using your left hand hold your right
    wrist to give some added support to
    your right arm. (fig. 1)

                OR

    Support your chin with both hands
    between forefinger and thumb.
    (fig. 2)

4.1 Open-close jaw movements: (fig. 3)

    Starting with your teeth touching,
    slowly let your jaw open towards
    your chest, against the resistance
    of your right hand. Move your jaw
    approximately the width of your
    index finger (i.e.) about 15 mm.
    Then allow your jaw to close slowly,
    also against the resistance of your
    hand.

4.2 Jaw movements to the side:

    Maintaining the arm support, slowly
    move your jaw to one side against
    the resistance of your hand, and
    then return to the starting position.
    Move your jaw to the other side
    against the resistance of your hand.

5. Repeat the open-close movement 20
    times, and the right and left
    movements 10 times in each direction.

    This sequence is carried out twice
    each day; once in the morning and
    once in the evening.

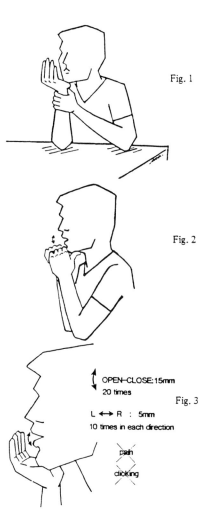

Fig. 1

Fig. 2

OPEN-CLOSE:15mm
20 times

L ⟷ R : 5mm
10 times in each direction

Fig. 3

pain

clicking

IMPORTANT POINTS :

1. Do not push your jaw forward; always open your jaw in an arc towards your
    chest.

2. Never open more than 20 mm; limit sideward movements to the left and
    right to about 5 mm.

3. Never perform the exercises so that pain or clicking sounds occur.

4. If you feel these exercises are causing an increase in discomfort, do not
    continue and contact the Clinic as soon as possible.

Index